Kick Cancer's Butt!

YOUR Journal for Kicking Cancer's Butt!!

Dianne Terry

Réalta Publications

Published by Réalta Publications in 2019

First Edition; First printing

Design and writing by Dianne Terry

ISBN: 978-1-950591-04-6

This Journal belongs to

If found, please call

In Case of Emergency, please call

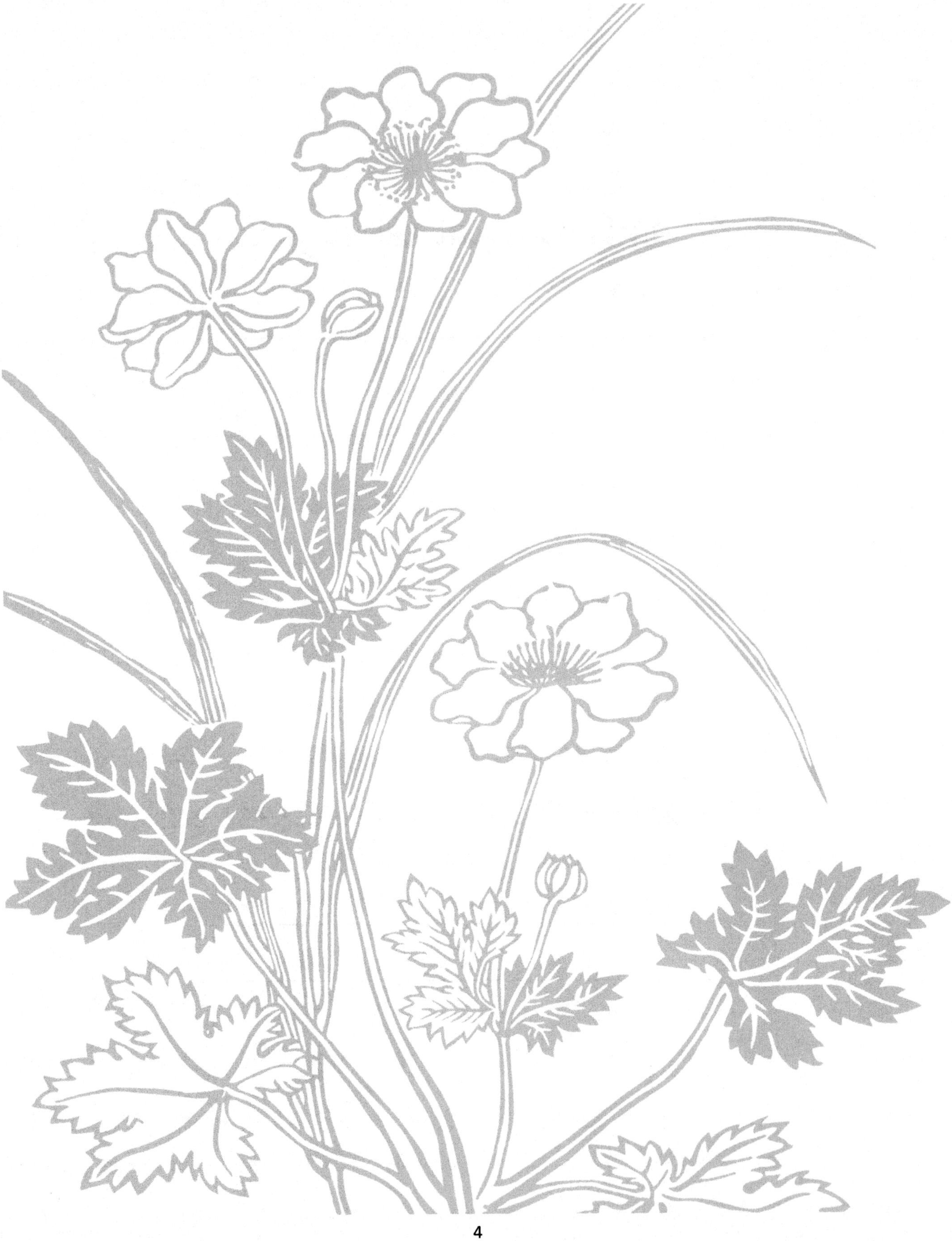

Dedication

This book is dedicated to all the people who have and will endure the seemingly endless treatments for the insidious disease called

CANCER.

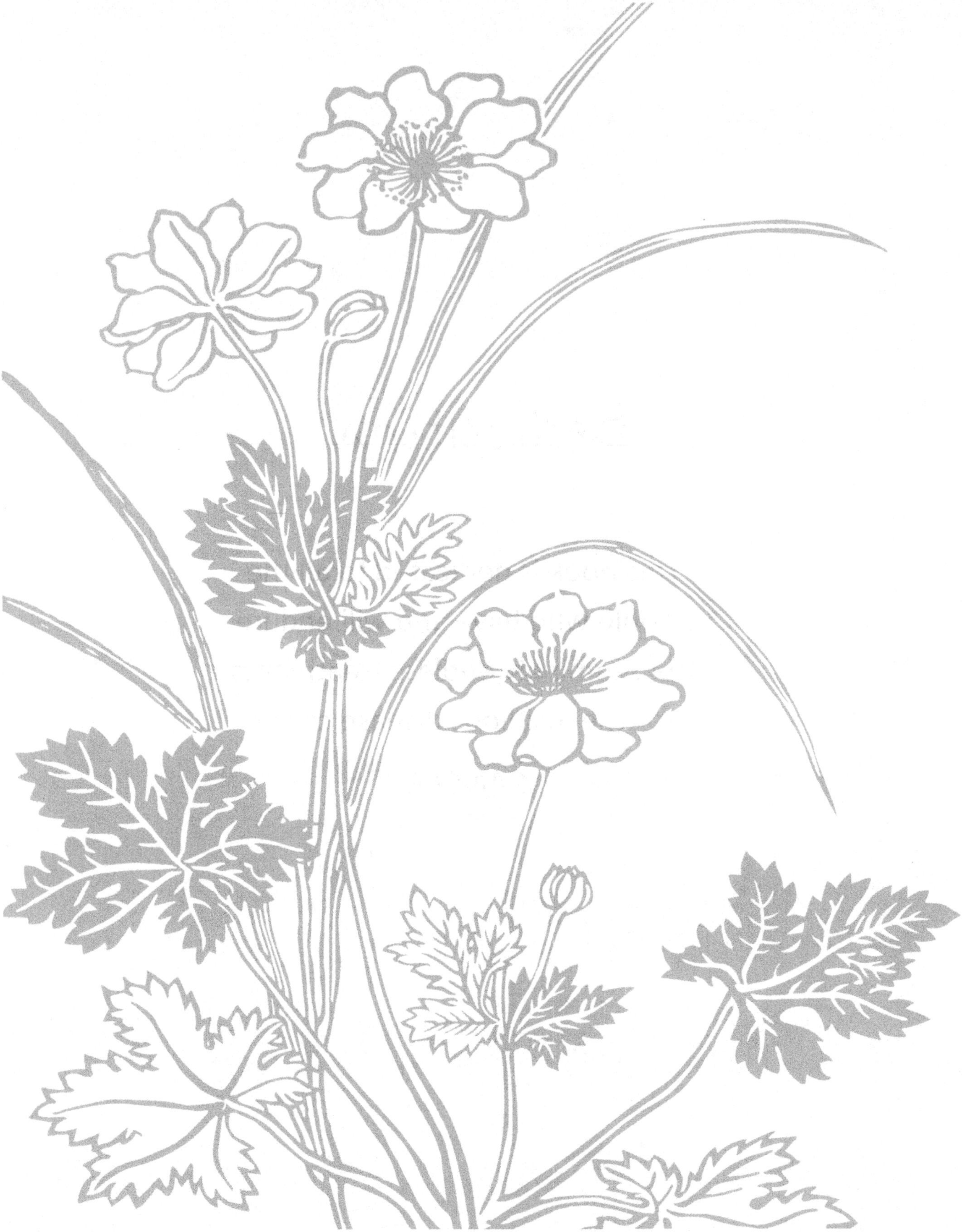

Table of Contents

A Personal Note to You

Hearing the words "You have CANCER" is probably one of the scariest, most devastating things you will ever experience. It feels like your heart actually stops beating in your chest for a moment. You may feel like crying or even screaming.

Thoughts of all the things you wanted to do but may not have time for now . . . You've been dreading hearing that word ever since you started down this road, even though you kept pushing it down—never saying "that word" out loud.

I can't take away your cancer, but I hope this journal will provide some resources and assurances for you. It is designed to help you capture important information about **you**: your health, your doctors, your visits for treatments, and especially how you **feel** during this journey from diagnosis to **cure**.

My sincere prayer and hope for you is this journal provides the "one-stop-shopping" you need as you embark on this journey. I'm not talking about the purchase of this journal—I'm talking about being able to corral everything you need to remember into one spot so you only have to pick up your journal as you get ready to head out the door to the next round of chemo or consultations.

One of the things we've noticed after dealing with cancer is "chemo brain" which seems to affect many if not all cancer patients. It's a fuzzy phenomenon that keeps you from being able to make sense of the simplest tasks. Perhaps it's just overwhelm, but more likely "chemo brain" is caused by the very treatment you are receiving. Because of this, it's hard to focus, be organized . . . and think of anything past survival.

It's hard to remember what you need to ask the doctor, what he tells you, special instructions about medications—so many things.

Whatever the cause for "chemo brain", simplifying your life is key to getting through all this and remaining sane. :)

Now, just so we're clear here—I'm not promising sanity, but if you keep things together *—as best you can—*and stay **positive**, you may find you are able to handle the ups and downs better.

> When you're dealing with cancer, a daily dose of inspiration may make a big difference in your outlook on life.

Keeping a positive outlook is proven to help with stress management, but when someone says to "think positive" or "be optimistic" during a time such as cancer, it can be much easier said than done.

I know cancer isn't all rainbow and butterflies and once you enter a dark mindset, it can be hard to get out of it. But most of us have that *one message* of hope and inspiration that somehow manages to help bring some perspective and optimism to the situation.

No one "deserves" cancer, and least of all you. So let's get started on this journey. On the next page, you will find instructions for how to get the best use of this journal.

How to Use This Journal

1. Commit to fighting this disease. Don't let it define you. FIGHT.
2. Don't fight alone. Enlist the help and support of your friends and family. They would be willing to take you to treatments when you don't feel like driving. They will pray with and for you. Take all the help you can get. Build your village with people who care about you.
3. Fill out the important information at the front of this journal as soon as you can. You will be using some of it at every appointment.
4. We all have a different path that leads us to the cancer diagnosis. Your story is important. Write about your journey to diagnosis. It may save the life of someone in your family some day—when they read about your first symptoms.
5. Important medical information is just that—fill out your blood type, medical alert, allergies and any surgeries you've had.
6. There are two pages for medical insurance—maybe too many for you, but fill in all applicable. Don't forget dental, eyeglasses, cancer insurance and anything else that comes to mind.
7. Medications—both prescriptions and over-the-counter vitamins and supplements. Your medical team will need all of this information to determine if anything you take affects or is affected by your prescribed treatments (chemo, etc.)
8. Write down all your doctors. It is important to have contact information for each of them so they can all be aware of your treatments. And yes, it is important for even your optometrist and dentist to be aware of what is going on with your health.
9. **Always** take this journal with you to doctor appointments or when going for treatments. By taking this along and keeping it up-to-date, you will have a record of all your questions, doctor instructions, blood tests . . . IN ONE PLACE.

How to Use This Journal (cont'd)

10. Capture your questions during the week to ask the doctor on your next visit. Then write down his responses and instructions.
11. Take time to write down how you feel each day—physically and emotionally.
12. Keep track of any side-effects you have to medications prescribed to you. Report those to the doctor when you see him next.
13. There's a year's worth of monthly calendar so you can keep track of important dates and events.
14. Two pages are provided for each doctor / treatment visit.
15. Twenty-six weeks of journaling is provided—one page for each week. Write about how you felt that day.
16. Twenty-six pages that include an inspirational saying and a picture are provided for encouragement. Take your coloring pencils along with you when you go for your appointments. It's the perfect way to relieve stress as you wait for an appointment or while receiving treatments.
17. Last . . . **but most important** . . . Be sure to focus on positives. Remember, even though chemo is running through your body, it is finding and attacking cancer cells—killing each one so it can no longer affect you.

This is how my journey began

I first noticed:

My first doctor's appointment:

The journey to diagnosis:

Diagnosis

My diagnosis was made on ___________________

When I heard the news, I felt _________________

____

____

____

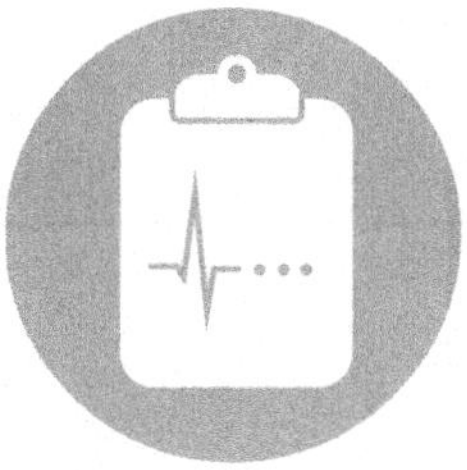

MY F.I.G.H.T. Plan

I realize that it's MY responsibility to fight this cancer growing inside me. Here are some things I will do to ensure victory:

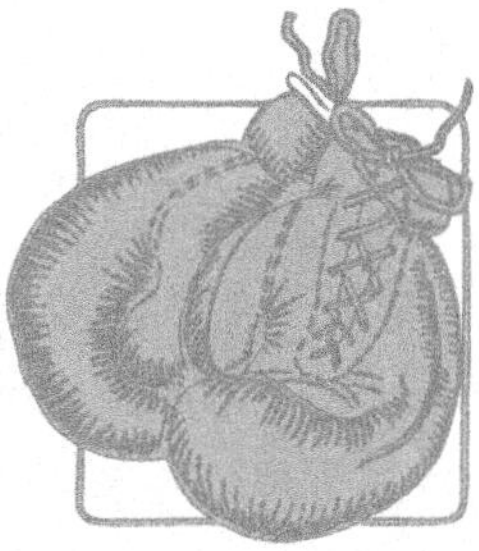

I. AM.

CANCER.FREE!!!!

Today's Date ________________

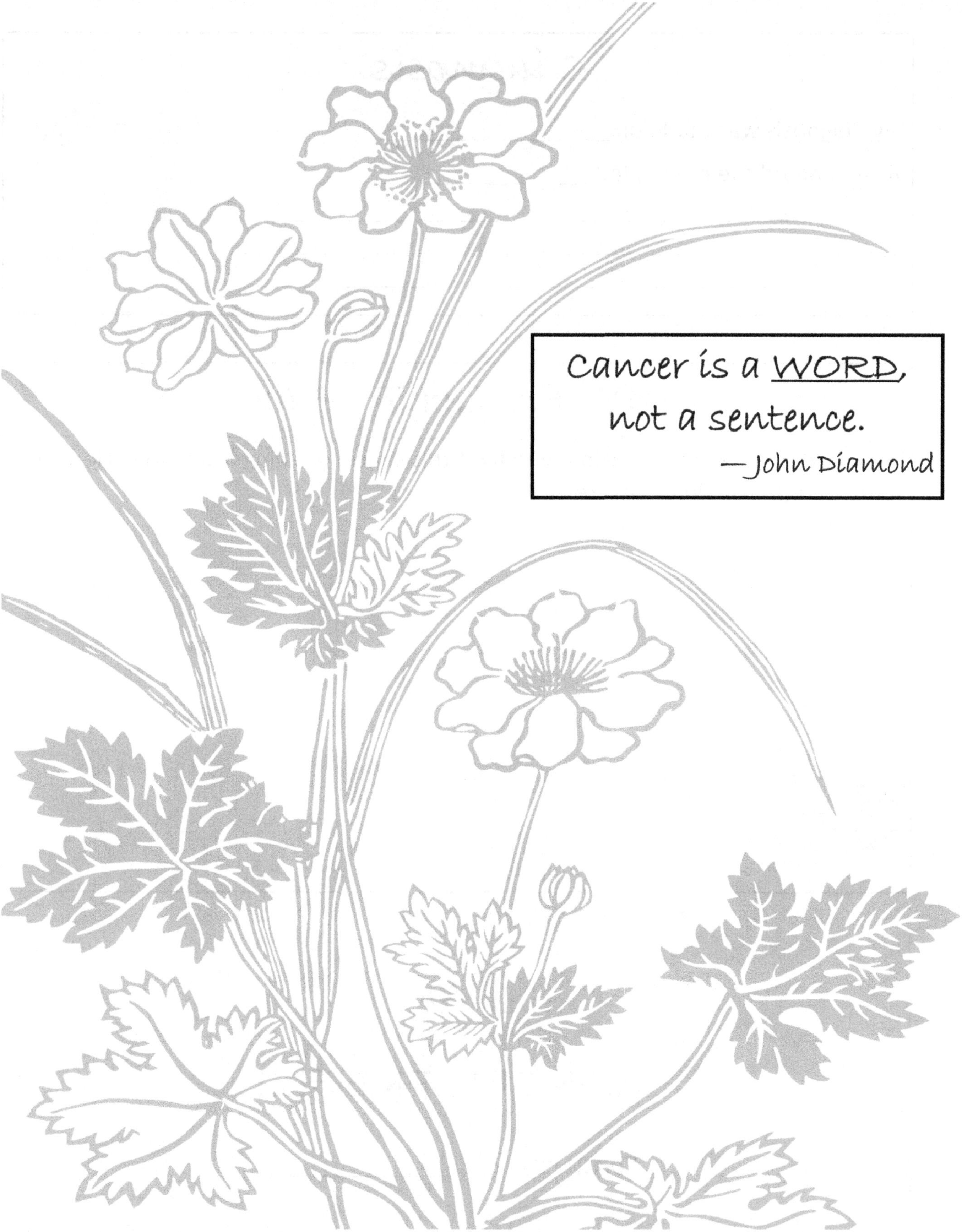

Cancer is a WORD, not a sentence.

—John Diamond

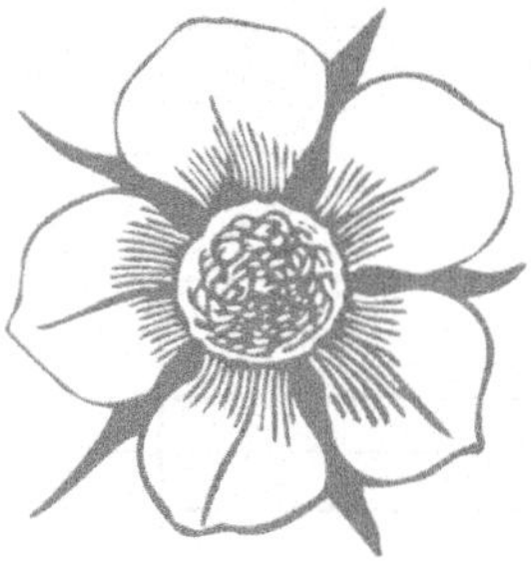

Important Medical Information

My Blood Type: ____________________

Medical Alert Information: ____________________

____

____

____

____

I am allergic to: ____________________

____

____

____

Previous Surgeries:

Date: ____________ Surgeon: ____________________
Surgery: ____________________

____

Date: ____________ Surgeon: ____________________
Surgery: ____________________

____

Date: ____________ Surgeon: ____________________
Surgery: ____________________

____

Date: ____________ Surgeon: ____________________
Surgery: ____________________

____

Date: ____________ Surgeon: ____________________
Surgery: ____________________

____

My Medical History

	Rheumatic Fever		Lung (Pulmonary Disease)
	Heart Disease		COPD
	Heart Attack >50		Water on the Lungs
	Heart Attack <50		Asthma
	High Blood Pressure		Type I Diabetes
	AFib—Atrial Fibrillation		Type II Diabetes
	Pacemaker		Type III Diabetes
	Heart Murmur		Hepatitis A, B, or C
	High Cholesterol		Headaches/Migraines (w/aura)
	Stroke		Headaches/Migraines (w/out aura)
	Whooping Cough (Pertussis)		Seizure Disorder
	Measles		Epilepsy
	Meningitis		Digestive Tract
	Chicken Pox (Varicella)		Gallbladder/Gallstones
	Mumps		Diabetes
	Pneumonia		Liver Disease / Hepatitis
	Polio		Thyroid
	Tuberculosis		Kidney Renal Disease
	HIV Infection		Kidney Stones
	Eczema		Prostate Problems
	Tattoo		Rheumatoid Arthritis
	Hay Fever		Prior Orthopedic Problems
	Hives (Uticaria)		Joint Problems
	Allergies		Depression / Suicide
	Ear/Nose/Throat		Alcoholism
	Hearing Problems		Drug Addiction
	Immune Disorder		Anxiety

My Medical History (cont'd)

	Skin Cancer		Panic Attacks
	Cancer		Mental Health Disorder
	Anemia		Fertility
	Hernia: Type ________________		Colon Polyps? ____
			Type: ____________________

My Family Medical History

Condition	* G/A/U C/P/S	Condition	* G/A/U C/P/S
Heart Disease		Cancer	
Heart Attack		Breast	
High Blood Pressure		Colorectal	
High Cholesterol		Lung	
Kidney Disease		Prostate / Ovarian	
Lung Disease		Skin	
Asthma		Other: ______________	
COPD		Liver Disease	
Migraines		Stroke	
Dementia		Tuberculosis	
Alzheimers		Depression/Suicide	
Mental Disorder		Epilepsy/Seizures	
Thyroid Disease		Diabetes	
Smokers		Alcoholism	
Osteoporosis		Drug Addiction	

Doctors and Hospitals

HOSPITAL: ______________________________
Address: ______________________________
____
City/State/Zip: ______________________________
Phone: ______________ Fax: ______________

PRIMARY CARE: ______________________________
Address: ______________________________
____
City/State/Zip: ______________________________
Phone: ______________ Fax: ______________

OB-GYN: ______________________________
Address: ______________________________
____
City/State/Zip: ______________________________
Phone: ______________ Fax: ______________

DENTIST: ______________________________
Address: ______________________________
____
City/State/Zip: ______________________________
Phone: ______________ Fax: ______________

OPTOMETRIST: ______________________________
Address: ______________________________
____
City/State/Zip: ______________________________
Phone: ______________ Fax: ______________

SPECIALIST: ______________________________
Address: ______________________________
____
City/State/Zip: ______________________________
Phone: ______________ Fax: ______________

Doctors and Hospitals

SPECIALIST: ______________________________
Address:______________________________
____
City/State/Zip:______________________________
Phone: ____________________ Fax: ____________________

SPECIALIST: ______________________________
Address:______________________________
____
City/State/Zip:______________________________
Phone: ____________________ Fax: ____________________

SPECIALIST: ______________________________
Address:______________________________
____
City/State/Zip:______________________________
Phone: ____________________ Fax: ____________________

SPECIALIST: ______________________________
Address:______________________________
____
City/State/Zip:______________________________
Phone: ____________________ Fax: ____________________

SPECIALIST: ______________________________
Address:______________________________
____
City/State/Zip:______________________________
Phone: ____________________ Fax: ____________________

SPECIALIST: ______________________________
Address:______________________________
____
City/State/Zip:______________________________
Phone: ____________________ Fax: ____________________

Medical Insurance

Primary Insurance: ______________________________
Policy #: ______________________________
Policy Start Date: ______________ **Policy End Date:** ______________
Address: ______________________________
City/State/Zip: ______________________________
Contact: ______________________________
Phone: ______________________________
Email: ______________________________

Secondary Insurance: ______________________________
Policy #: ______________________________
Policy Start Date: ______________ **Policy End Date:** ______________
Address: ______________________________
City/State/Zip: ______________________________
Contact: ______________________________
Phone: ______________________________
Email: ______________________________

Additional Insurance: ______________________________
Policy #: ______________________________
Policy Start Date: ______________ **Policy End Date:** ______________
Address: ______________________________
City/State/Zip: ______________________________
Contact: ______________________________
Phone: ______________________________
Email: ______________________________

Additional Insurance: ______________________________
Policy #: ______________________________
Policy Start Date: ______________ **Policy End Date:** ______________
Address: ______________________________
City/State/Zip: ______________________________
Contact: ______________________________
Phone: ______________________________
Email: ______________________________

Additional Medical Insurance

Additional Insurance: ______________________________
Policy #: ______________________________
Policy Start Date:______________ Policy End Date:______________
Address: ______________________________
City/State/Zip: ______________________________
Contact: ______________________________
Phone: ______________________________
Email:______________________________

Additional Insurance: ______________________________
Policy #: ______________________________
Policy Start Date:______________ Policy End Date:______________
Address: ______________________________
City/State/Zip: ______________________________
Contact: ______________________________
Phone: ______________________________
Email:______________________________

Additional Insurance: ______________________________
Policy #: ______________________________
Policy Start Date:______________ Policy End Date:______________
Address: ______________________________
City/State/Zip: ______________________________
Contact: ______________________________
Phone: ______________________________
Email:______________________________

Additional Insurance: ______________________________
Policy #: ______________________________
Policy Start Date:______________ Policy End Date:______________
Address: ______________________________
City/State/Zip: ______________________________
Contact: ______________________________
Phone: ______________________________
Email:______________________________

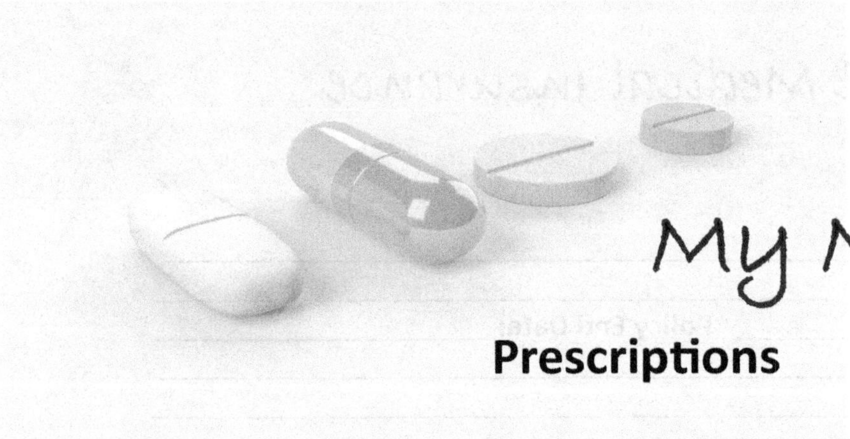

My Medications

Prescriptions

Name	Dosage	Frequency	What's it For?

My Medications

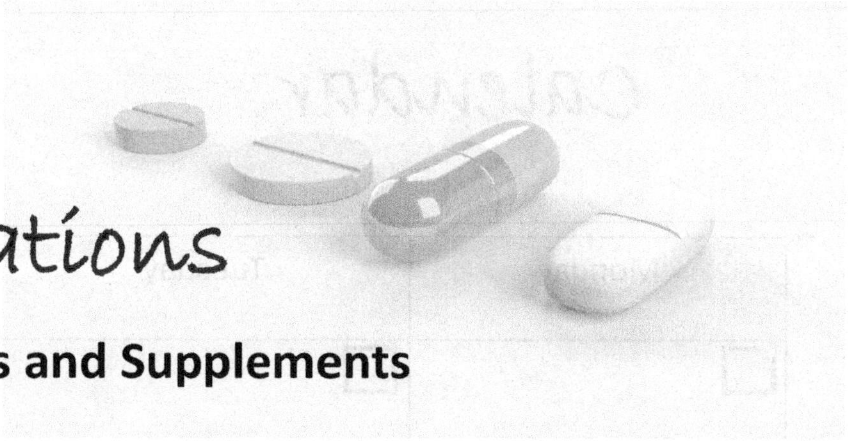

Vitamins and Supplements

Name	Dosage	Frequency	What's it For?

Calendar

Year: _______

Monday	Tuesday	Wednesday
☐	☐	☐
☐	☐	☐
☐	☐	☐
☐	☐	☐
☐	☐	☐

Notes: ____

Calendar

Month: ____________________

Thursday	Friday	Saturday / Sunday
☐	☐	☐ / ☐
☐	☐	☐ / ☐
☐	☐	☐ / ☐
☐	☐	☐ / ☐
☐	☐	☐ / ☐

Notes: ____________________

Calendar

Year: ________

Monday	Tuesday	Wednesday
☐	☐	☐
☐	☐	☐
☐	☐	☐
☐	☐	☐
☐	☐	☐

Notes: ____

Calendar

Month: ______________________

Thursday	Friday	Saturday / Sunday
☐	☐	☐ / ☐
☐	☐	☐ / ☐
☐	☐	☐ / ☐
☐	☐	☐ / ☐
☐	☐	☐ / ☐

Notes: ______________________

Calendar

Year: ________

Monday	Tuesday	Wednesday
☐	☐	☐
☐	☐	☐
☐	☐	☐
☐	☐	☐
☐	☐	☐

Notes: ________________________________

Calendar

Month: ______________________

Thursday	Friday	Saturday / Sunday
☐	☐	☐ / ☐
☐	☐	☐ / ☐
☐	☐	☐ / ☐
☐	☐	☐ / ☐
☐	☐	☐ / ☐

Notes: ______________________

Calendar

Year: ________

Monday	Tuesday	Wednesday
☐	☐	☐
☐	☐	☐
☐	☐	☐
☐	☐	☐
☐	☐	☐

Notes: ______________________________

Calendar

Month: ____________________

Thursday	Friday	Saturday / Sunday
☐	☐	☐ / ☐
☐	☐	☐ / ☐
☐	☐	☐ / ☐
☐	☐	☐ / ☐
☐	☐	☐ / ☐

Notes: ____________________

Calendar

Year: ______

Monday	Tuesday	Wednesday
☐	☐	☐
☐	☐	☐
☐	☐	☐
☐	☐	☐
☐	☐	☐

Notes: ______

Calendar

Month: ______________________

Thursday	Friday	Saturday / Sunday
☐	☐	☐ / ☐
☐	☐	☐ / ☐
☐	☐	☐ / ☐
☐	☐	☐ / ☐
☐	☐	☐ / ☐

Notes: ______________________

Calendar

Year: ________

Monday	Tuesday	Wednesday
☐	☐	☐
☐	☐	☐
☐	☐	☐
☐	☐	☐
☐	☐	☐

Notes: ____

____

____

____

____

____

____

____

Calendar

Month: ______________________

Thursday	Friday	Saturday / Sunday
☐	☐	☐ / ☐
☐	☐	☐ / ☐
☐	☐	☐ / ☐
☐	☐	☐ / ☐
☐	☐	☐ / ☐

Notes: ______________________

Calendar

Year: ________

Monday	Tuesday	Wednesday
☐	☐	☐
☐	☐	☐
☐	☐	☐
☐	☐	☐
☐	☐	☐

Notes: ____

Calendar

Month: ______________________

Thursday	Friday	Saturday / Sunday
☐	☐	☐ / ☐
☐	☐	☐ / ☐
☐	☐	☐ / ☐
☐	☐	☐ / ☐
☐	☐	☐ / ☐

Notes: ______________________

Calendar

Year: ________

Monday	Tuesday	Wednesday
☐	☐	☐
☐	☐	☐
☐	☐	☐
☐	☐	☐
☐	☐	☐

Notes: ____

Calendar

Month: ____________________

Thursday	Friday	Saturday / Sunday
☐	☐	☐ / ☐
☐	☐	☐ / ☐
☐	☐	☐ / ☐
☐	☐	☐ / ☐
☐	☐	☐ / ☐

Notes: ____________________

Calendar

Year: ________

Monday	Tuesday	Wednesday
☐	☐	☐
☐	☐	☐
☐	☐	☐
☐	☐	☐
☐	☐	☐

Notes: ____

Calendar

Month: ______________________

Thursday	Friday	Saturday / Sunday
☐	☐	☐ / ☐
☐	☐	☐ / ☐
☐	☐	☐ / ☐
☐	☐	☐ / ☐
☐	☐	☐ / ☐

Notes: ______________________

Calendar

Year: ________

Monday	Tuesday	Wednesday
☐	☐	☐
☐	☐	☐
☐	☐	☐
☐	☐	☐
☐	☐	☐

Notes: ____

Calendar

Month: ______________________

Thursday	Friday	Saturday / Sunday
☐	☐	☐ / ☐
☐	☐	☐ / ☐
☐	☐	☐ / ☐
☐	☐	☐ / ☐
☐	☐	☐ / ☐

Notes: ______________________

Calendar

Year: ________

Monday	Tuesday	Wednesday
☐	☐	☐
☐	☐	☐
☐	☐	☐
☐	☐	☐
☐	☐	☐

Notes: ____________________

Calendar

Month: ______________________

Thursday	Friday	Saturday / Sunday
☐	☐	☐ / ☐
☐	☐	☐ / ☐
☐	☐	☐ / ☐
☐	☐	☐ / ☐
☐	☐	☐ / ☐

Notes: ______________________

Calendar

Year: ________

Monday	Tuesday	Wednesday
☐	☐	☐
☐	☐	☐
☐	☐	☐
☐	☐	☐
☐	☐	☐

Notes: ____

Calendar

Month: ____________________

Thursday	Friday	Saturday / Sunday
☐	☐	☐ / ☐
☐	☐	☐ / ☐
☐	☐	☐ / ☐
☐	☐	☐ / ☐
☐	☐	☐ / ☐

Notes: ____________________

Office Visit

Date/Time: ______________________________

Doctor: ______________________________

Reason for Visit: ____

Blood Cell Count

White Blood Cell	Red Blood Cell
Hemoglobin	Hematocrit
Platelets	Other

Questions to ask the doctor: ____

____

____

____

____

____

____

Doctor's Diagnosis/Feedback: ____

____

____

____

____

Treatment Received Today: ____

____

____

Any medication changes? ____

____

____

Office Visit

Next Visit

Date/Time ____

Purpose ____

Who will I see? ____

Today I'm feeling:

- O Better
- O Worse
- O Same
- O Pain
- O Fatigue
- O Depression

NOTES

Office Visit

Date/Time: ______________________

Doctor: ______________________

Reason for Visit: ______________________

Blood Cell Count

White Blood Cell	Red Blood Cell
Hemoglobin	Hematocrit
Platelets	Other

Questions to ask the doctor: ______________________

Doctor's Diagnosis/Feedback: ______________________

Treatment Received Today: ______________________

Any medication changes? ______________________

Office Visit

Next Visit

Date/Time ____

Purpose ____

Who will I see? ____

Today I'm feeling:

- O Better
- O Worse
- O Same
- O Pain
- O Fatigue
- O Depression

NOTES

Office Visit

Date/Time: ______________________________

Doctor: ______________________________

Reason for Visit: ____

Blood Cell Count

White Blood Cell	Red Blood Cell
Hemoglobin	Hematocrit
Platelets	Other

Questions to ask the doctor: ____

Doctor's Diagnosis/Feedback: ____

Treatment Received Today: ____

Any medication changes? ____

Office Visit

Next Visit

Date/Time ______________________________

Purpose ______________________________

Who will I see? ______________________________

Today I'm feeling:

- O Better
- O Worse
- O Same
- O Pain
- O Fatigue
- O Depression

NOTES

Office Visit

Date/Time: ______________________________

Doctor: ______________________________

Reason for Visit: ______________________________

Blood Cell Count

White Blood Cell	Red Blood Cell
Hemoglobin	Hematocrit
Platelets	Other

Questions to ask the doctor: ______________________________

Doctor's Diagnosis/Feedback: ______________________________

Treatment Received Today: ______________________________

Any medication changes? ______________________________

Office Visit

Next Visit

Date/Time ______________________________

Purpose ______________________________

Who will I see? ______________________________

Today I'm feeling:

- O Better
- O Worse
- O Same
- O Pain
- O Fatigue
- O Depression

NOTES

Office Visit

Date/Time: ______________________________

Doctor: ______________________________

Reason for Visit: ____

Blood Cell Count

White Blood Cell	Red Blood Cell
Hemoglobin	Hematocrit
Platelets	Other

Questions to ask the doctor: ____

____

____

____

____

____

____

Doctor's Diagnosis/Feedback: ____

____

____

____

____

Treatment Received Today: ____

____

____

Any medication changes? ____

____

____

Office Visit

Next Visit

Date/Time ____

Purpose ____

Who will I see? ____

Today I'm feeling:

- O Better
- O Worse
- O Same
- O Pain
- O Fatigue
- O Depression

NOTES

Office Visit

Date/Time: ______________________________

Doctor: ______________________________

Reason for Visit: ____

Blood Cell Count

White Blood Cell	Red Blood Cell
Hemoglobin	Hematocrit
Platelets	Other

Questions to ask the doctor: ____

____

____

____

____

____

____

Doctor's Diagnosis/Feedback: ____

____

____

____

____

Treatment Received Today: ____

____

____

Any medication changes? ____

____

____

Office Visit

Next Visit

Date/Time ______________________________

Purpose ______________________________

Who will I see? ______________________________

Today I'm feeling:

- O Better
- O Worse
- O Same
- O Pain
- O Fatigue
- O Depression

NOTES

Office Visit

Date/Time: ______________________

Doctor: ______________________

Reason for Visit: ______________________

Blood Cell Count

White Blood Cell	Red Blood Cell
Hemoglobin	Hematocrit
Platelets	Other

Questions to ask the doctor: ______________________

Doctor's Diagnosis/Feedback: ______________________

Treatment Received Today: ______________________

Any medication changes? ______________________

Office Visit

Next Visit

Date/Time ____________________

Purpose ____________________

Who will I see? ____________________

Today I'm feeling:

- O Better
- O Worse
- O Same
- O Pain
- O Fatigue
- O Depression

NOTES

Office Visit

Date/Time: ______________________________

Doctor: ______________________________

Reason for Visit: ______________________________

Blood Cell Count

White Blood Cell	Red Blood Cell
Hemoglobin	Hematocrit
Platelets	Other

Questions to ask the doctor: ______________________________

Doctor's Diagnosis/Feedback: ______________________________

Treatment Received Today: ______________________________

Any medication changes? ______________________________

Office Visit

Next Visit

Date/Time ______________________________

Purpose ______________________________

Who will I see? ______________________________

Today I'm feeling:

- O Better
- O Worse
- O Same
- O Pain
- O Fatigue
- O Depression

NOTES

Office Visit

Date/Time: ______________________________

Doctor: ______________________________

Reason for Visit: ____

Blood Cell Count

White Blood Cell	Red Blood Cell
Hemoglobin	Hematocrit
Platelets	Other

Questions to ask the doctor: ____

____

____

____

____

____

____

Doctor's Diagnosis/Feedback: ____

____

____

____

____

Treatment Received Today: ____

____

____

Any medication changes? ____

____

____

Office Visit

Next Visit

Date/Time ____

Purpose ____

Who will I see? _____________________________________

Today I'm feeling:

- O Better
- O Worse
- O Same
- O Pain
- O Fatigue
- O Depression

NOTES

Office Visit

Date/Time: ______________________________

Doctor: ______________________________

Reason for Visit: ____

Blood Cell Count

White Blood Cell	Red Blood Cell
Hemoglobin	Hematocrit
Platelets	Other

Questions to ask the doctor: ____

____

____

____

____

____

____

Doctor's Diagnosis/Feedback: ____

____

____

____

____

Treatment Received Today: ____

____

____

Any medication changes? ____

____

____

Office Visit

Next Visit

Date/Time ____

Purpose ____

Who will I see? ______________________________________

Today I'm feeling:

- O Better
- O Worse
- O Same
- O Pain
- O Fatigue
- O Depression

NOTES

Office Visit

Date/Time: ______________________________

Doctor: ______________________________

Reason for Visit: ______________________________

Blood Cell Count

White Blood Cell	Red Blood Cell
Hemoglobin	Hematocrit
Platelets	Other

Questions to ask the doctor: ______________________________

Doctor's Diagnosis/Feedback: ______________________________

Treatment Received Today: ______________________________

Any medication changes? ______________________________

Office Visit

Next Visit

Date/Time ____

Purpose ____

Who will I see? ____

Today I'm feeling:

- O Better
- O Worse
- O Same
- O Pain
- O Fatigue
- O Depression

NOTES

Office Visit

Date/Time: ____________________

Doctor: ____________________

Reason for Visit: ____________________

Blood Cell Count

White Blood Cell	Red Blood Cell
Hemoglobin	Hematocrit
Platelets	Other

Questions to ask the doctor: ____________________

Doctor's Diagnosis/Feedback: ____________________

Treatment Received Today: ____________________

Any medication changes? ____________________

Office Visit

Next Visit

Date/Time ____

Purpose ____

Who will I see? _______________________________________

Today I'm feeling:

- O Better
- O Worse
- O Same
- O Pain
- O Fatigue
- O Depression

NOTES

Office Visit

Date/Time: ____________________

Doctor: ____________________

Reason for Visit: ____________________

Blood Cell Count

White Blood Cell	Red Blood Cell
Hemoglobin	Hematocrit
Platelets	Other

Questions to ask the doctor: ____________________

Doctor's Diagnosis/Feedback: ____________________

Treatment Received Today: ____________________

Any medication changes? ____________________

Office Visit

Next Visit

Date/Time ______________________________

Purpose ______________________________

Who will I see? ______________________________

Today I'm feeling:

- O Better
- O Worse
- O Same
- O Pain
- O Fatigue
- O Depression

NOTES

Office Visit

Date/Time: ______________________________

Doctor: ______________________________

Reason for Visit: ____

Blood Cell Count

White Blood Cell	Red Blood Cell
Hemoglobin	Hematocrit
Platelets	Other

Questions to ask the doctor: ____

____

____

____

____

____

____

Doctor's Diagnosis/Feedback: ____

____

____

____

____

Treatment Received Today: ____

____

____

Any medication changes? ____

____

____

Office Visit

Next Visit

Date/Time ______________________________

Purpose ______________________________

Who will I see? ______________________________

Today I'm feeling:

- O Better
- O Worse
- O Same
- O Pain
- O Fatigue
- O Depression

NOTES

Office Visit

Date/Time: ______________________

Doctor: ______________________

Reason for Visit: ______________________

Blood Cell Count

White Blood Cell	Red Blood Cell
Hemoglobin	Hematocrit
Platelets	Other

Questions to ask the doctor: ______________________

Doctor's Diagnosis/Feedback: ______________________

Treatment Received Today: ______________________

Any medication changes? ______________________

Office Visit

Next Visit

Date/Time ____

Purpose ____

Who will I see? ____

Today I'm feeling:

- O Better
- O Worse
- O Same
- O Pain
- O Fatigue
- O Depression

NOTES

Office Visit

Date/Time: ______________________________

Doctor: ________________________________

Reason for Visit: ____

Blood Cell Count

White Blood Cell	Red Blood Cell
Hemoglobin	Hematocrit
Platelets	Other

Questions to ask the doctor: ______________________________________

Doctor's Diagnosis/Feedback: ______________________________________

Treatment Received Today: ____

Any medication changes? ____

Office Visit

Next Visit

Date/Time ______________________________

Purpose ______________________________

Who will I see? ______________________________

Today I'm feeling:

- O Better
- O Worse
- O Same
- O Pain
- O Fatigue
- O Depression

NOTES

Office Visit

Date/Time: ______________________________

Doctor: ________________________________

Reason for Visit: ____

Blood Cell Count

White Blood Cell	Red Blood Cell
Hemoglobin	Hematocrit
Platelets	Other

Questions to ask the doctor: ____

____

____

____

____

____

____

Doctor's Diagnosis/Feedback: ____

____

____

____

____

Treatment Received Today: ____

____

____

Any medication changes? ____

____

____

Office Visit

Next Visit

Date/Time ____

Purpose ____

Who will I see? ____

Today I'm feeling:

- O Better
- O Worse
- O Same
- O Pain
- O Fatigue
- O Depression

NOTES

Office Visit

Date/Time: ____________________

Doctor: ____________________

Reason for Visit: ____________________

Blood Cell Count

White Blood Cell	Red Blood Cell
Hemoglobin	Hematocrit
Platelets	Other

Questions to ask the doctor: ____________________

Doctor's Diagnosis/Feedback: ____________________

Treatment Received Today: ____________________

Any medication changes? ____________________

Office Visit

Next Visit

Date/Time ____

Purpose ____

Who will I see? ____

Today I'm feeling:

- O Better
- O Worse
- O Same
- O Pain
- O Fatigue
- O Depression

NOTES

Office Visit

Date/Time: ______________________________

Doctor: ________________________________

Reason for Visit: ____

Blood Cell Count

White Blood Cell	Red Blood Cell
Hemoglobin	Hematocrit
Platelets	Other

Questions to ask the doctor: ____

Doctor's Diagnosis/Feedback: ____

Treatment Received Today: ____

Any medication changes? ____

Office Visit

Next Visit

Date/Time ______________________________

Purpose ______________________________

Who will I see? ______________________________

Today I'm feeling:

- O Better
- O Worse
- O Same
- O Pain
- O Fatigue
- O Depression

NOTES

Office Visit

Date/Time: ______________________

Doctor: ______________________

Reason for Visit: ______________________

Blood Cell Count

White Blood Cell	Red Blood Cell
Hemoglobin	Hematocrit
Platelets	Other

Questions to ask the doctor: ______________________

____

____

____

____

____

____

Doctor's Diagnosis/Feedback: ______________________

____

____

____

____

Treatment Received Today: ______________________

____

____

Any medication changes? ______________________

____

____

Office Visit

Next Visit

Date/Time ______________________________

Purpose ______________________________

Who will I see? ______________________________

Today I'm feeling:

- O Better
- O Worse
- O Same
- O Pain
- O Fatigue
- O Depression

NOTES

Office Visit

Date/Time: ______________________________

Doctor: ______________________________

Reason for Visit: ______________________________

Blood Cell Count

White Blood Cell	Red Blood Cell
Hemoglobin	Hematocrit
Platelets	Other

Questions to ask the doctor: ______________________________

____

____

____

____

____

____

Doctor's Diagnosis/Feedback: ______________________________

____

____

____

____

Treatment Received Today: ______________________________

____

____

Any medication changes? ______________________________

____

____

Office Visit

Next Visit

Date/Time ______________________________

Purpose ______________________________

Who will I see? ______________________________

Today I'm feeling:

- O Better
- O Worse
- O Same
- O Pain
- O Fatigue
- O Depression

NOTES

Office Visit

Date/Time: ______________________________

Doctor: _________________________________

Reason for Visit: ____

Blood Cell Count

White Blood Cell	Red Blood Cell
Hemoglobin	Hematocrit
Platelets	Other

Questions to ask the doctor: ____

Doctor's Diagnosis/Feedback: ____

Treatment Received Today: ____

Any medication changes? ____

Office Visit

Next Visit

Date/Time ____

Purpose ____

Who will I see? ____

Today I'm feeling:

- O Better
- O Worse
- O Same
- O Pain
- O Fatigue
- O Depression

NOTES

Office Visit

Date/Time: ______________________________

Doctor: ______________________________

Reason for Visit: ____

Blood Cell Count

White Blood Cell	Red Blood Cell
Hemoglobin	Hematocrit
Platelets	Other

Questions to ask the doctor: ____

Doctor's Diagnosis/Feedback: ____

Treatment Received Today: ____

Any medication changes? ____

Office Visit

Next Visit

Date/Time ____________________

Purpose ____________________

Who will I see? ____________________

Today I'm feeling:

- O Better
- O Worse
- O Same
- O Pain
- O Fatigue
- O Depression

NOTES

Office Visit

Date/Time: ______________________________

Doctor: ______________________________

Reason for Visit: ______________________________

Blood Cell Count

White Blood Cell	Red Blood Cell
Hemoglobin	Hematocrit
Platelets	Other

Questions to ask the doctor: ______________________________

Doctor's Diagnosis/Feedback: ______________________________

Treatment Received Today: ______________________________

Any medication changes? ______________________________

Office Visit

Next Visit

Date/Time ____

Purpose ____

Who will I see? _______________________________________

Today I'm feeling:

- O Better
- O Worse
- O Same
- O Pain
- O Fatigue
- O Depression

NOTES

Office Visit

Date/Time: ______________________________

Doctor: ______________________________

Reason for Visit: ____

Blood Cell Count

White Blood Cell	Red Blood Cell
Hemoglobin	Hematocrit
Platelets	Other

Questions to ask the doctor: ____

____

____

____

____

____

____

Doctor's Diagnosis/Feedback: ____

____

____

____

____

Treatment Received Today: ____

____

____

Any medication changes? ____

____

____

Office Visit

Next Visit

Date/Time ______________________________

Purpose ______________________________

Who will I see? ______________________________

Today I'm feeling:

- O Better
- O Worse
- O Same
- O Pain
- O Fatigue
- O Depression

NOTES

Office Visit

Date/Time: ______________________________

Doctor: ______________________________

Reason for Visit: ____

Blood Cell Count

White Blood Cell	Red Blood Cell
Hemoglobin	Hematocrit
Platelets	Other

Questions to ask the doctor: ____

Doctor's Diagnosis/Feedback: ____

Treatment Received Today: ____

Any medication changes? ____

Office Visit

Next Visit

Date/Time ______________________________

Purpose ______________________________

Who will I see? ______________________________

Today I'm feeling:

- O Better
- O Worse
- O Same
- O Pain
- O Fatigue
- O Depression

NOTES

My Journal

Week of ______________________

Monday

Tuesday

Wednesday

Thursday

My Journal

Friday

Saturday

Sunday

Notes

My Journal

Week of ____________________

Monday

Tuesday

Wednesday

Thursday

My Journal

Friday

Saturday

Sunday

Notes

My Journal

Week of ____________________

Monday

Tuesday

Wednesday

Thursday

My Journal

Friday

Saturday

Sunday

Notes

My Journal

Week of ____________________

Monday

Tuesday

Wednesday

Thursday

My Journal

Friday

Saturday

Sunday

Notes

My Journal

Week of ______________________

Monday

Tuesday

Wednesday

Thursday

My Journal

Friday

Saturday

Sunday

Notes

My Journal

Week of ______________________

Monday

Tuesday

Wednesday

Thursday

My Journal

Friday

Saturday

Sunday

Notes

My Journal

Week of ____________________

Monday

Tuesday

Wednesday

Thursday

My Journal

Friday

Saturday

Sunday

Notes

My Journal

Week of ____________________

Monday

Tuesday

Wednesday

Thursday

My Journal

Friday

Saturday

Sunday

Notes

My Journal

Week of ______________________

Monday

Tuesday

Wednesday

Thursday

My Journal

Friday

Saturday

Sunday

Notes

My Journal

Week of ___________________________

Monday

Tuesday

Wednesday

Thursday

My Journal

Friday

Saturday

Sunday

Notes

My Journal

Week of ______________________

Monday

Tuesday

Wednesday

Thursday

My Journal

Friday

Saturday

Sunday

Notes

My Journal

Week of ____________________

Monday

Tuesday

Wednesday

Thursday

My Journal

Friday

Saturday

Sunday

Notes

My Journal

Week of ______________________

Monday

Tuesday

Wednesday

Thursday

My Journal

Friday

Saturday

Sunday

Notes

My Journal

Week of ______________________

Monday

Tuesday

Wednesday

Thursday

My Journal

Friday

Saturday

Sunday

Notes

My Journal

Week of ______________________

Monday

Tuesday

Wednesday

Thursday

My Journal

Friday

Saturday

Sunday

Notes

My Journal

Week of ____________________

Monday

Tuesday

Wednesday

Thursday

My Journal

Friday

Saturday

Sunday

Notes

My Journal

Week of ______________________

Monday

Tuesday

Wednesday

Thursday

My Journal

Friday

Saturday

Sunday

Notes

My Journal

Week of ____________________

Monday

Tuesday

Wednesday

Thursday

My Journal

Friday

Saturday

Sunday

Notes

My Journal

Week of ______________________

Monday

Tuesday

Wednesday

Thursday

My Journal

Friday

Saturday

Sunday

Notes

My Journal

Week of ____________________

Monday

Tuesday

Wednesday

Thursday

My Journal

Friday

Saturday

Sunday

Notes

My Journal

Week of ____________________

Monday

Tuesday

Wednesday

Thursday

My Journal

Friday

Saturday

Sunday

Notes

My Journal

Week of ____________________

Monday

Tuesday

Wednesday

Thursday

My Journal

Friday

Saturday

Sunday

Notes

My Journal

Week of ______________________

Monday

Tuesday

Wednesday

Thursday

My Journal

Friday

Saturday

Sunday

Notes

My Journal

Week of ____________________

Monday

Tuesday

Wednesday

Thursday

My Journal

Friday

Saturday

Sunday

Notes

My Journal

Week of ______________________

Monday

Tuesday

Wednesday

Thursday

My Journal

Friday

Saturday

Sunday

Notes

My Journal

Week of ______________________

Monday

Tuesday

Wednesday

Thursday

My Journal

Friday

Saturday

Sunday

Notes

My Journal

Week of ____________________

Monday

Tuesday

Wednesday

Thursday

My Journal

Friday

Saturday

Sunday

Notes

Above all, cancer is a spiritual practice that teaches me about faith and resilience.

– Kris Carr

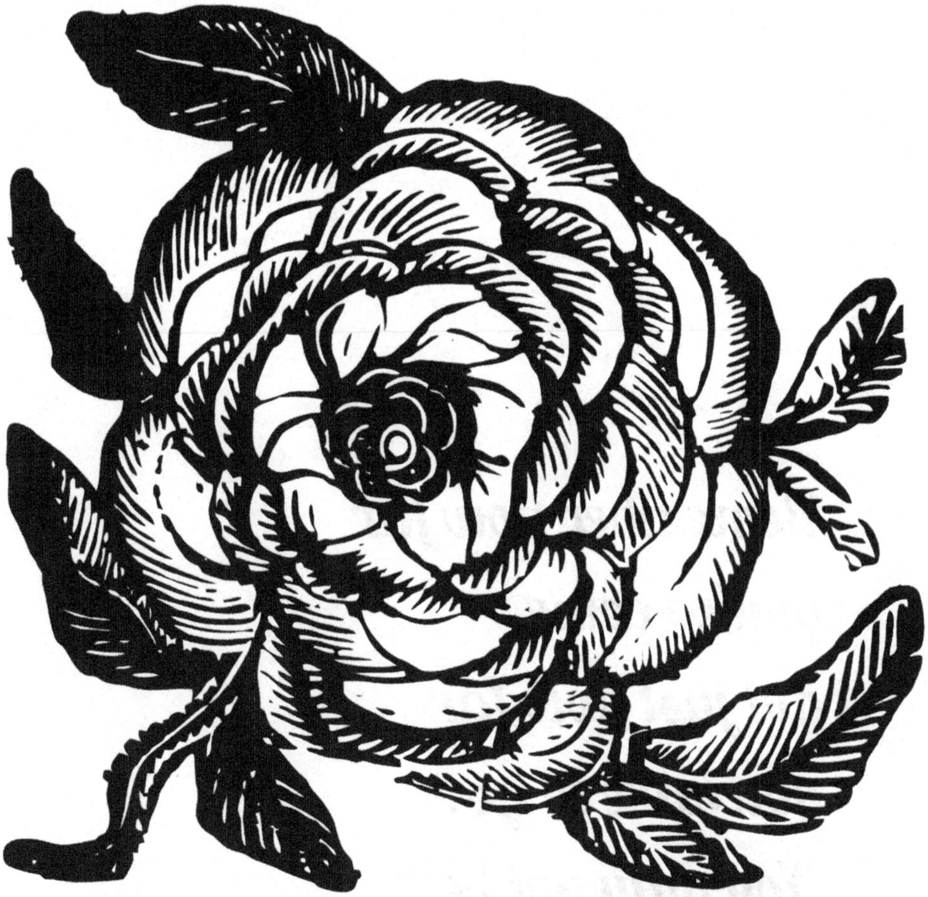

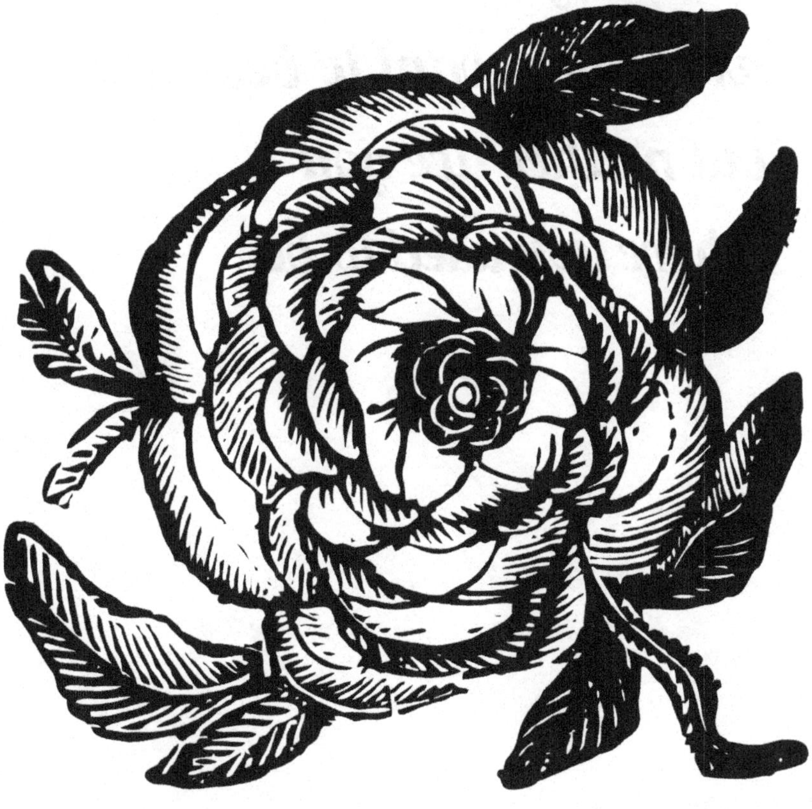

Remember how far
you've come,
not just how far
you have to go.
You may not be
where you want to be,
but neither are you
where you used to be.

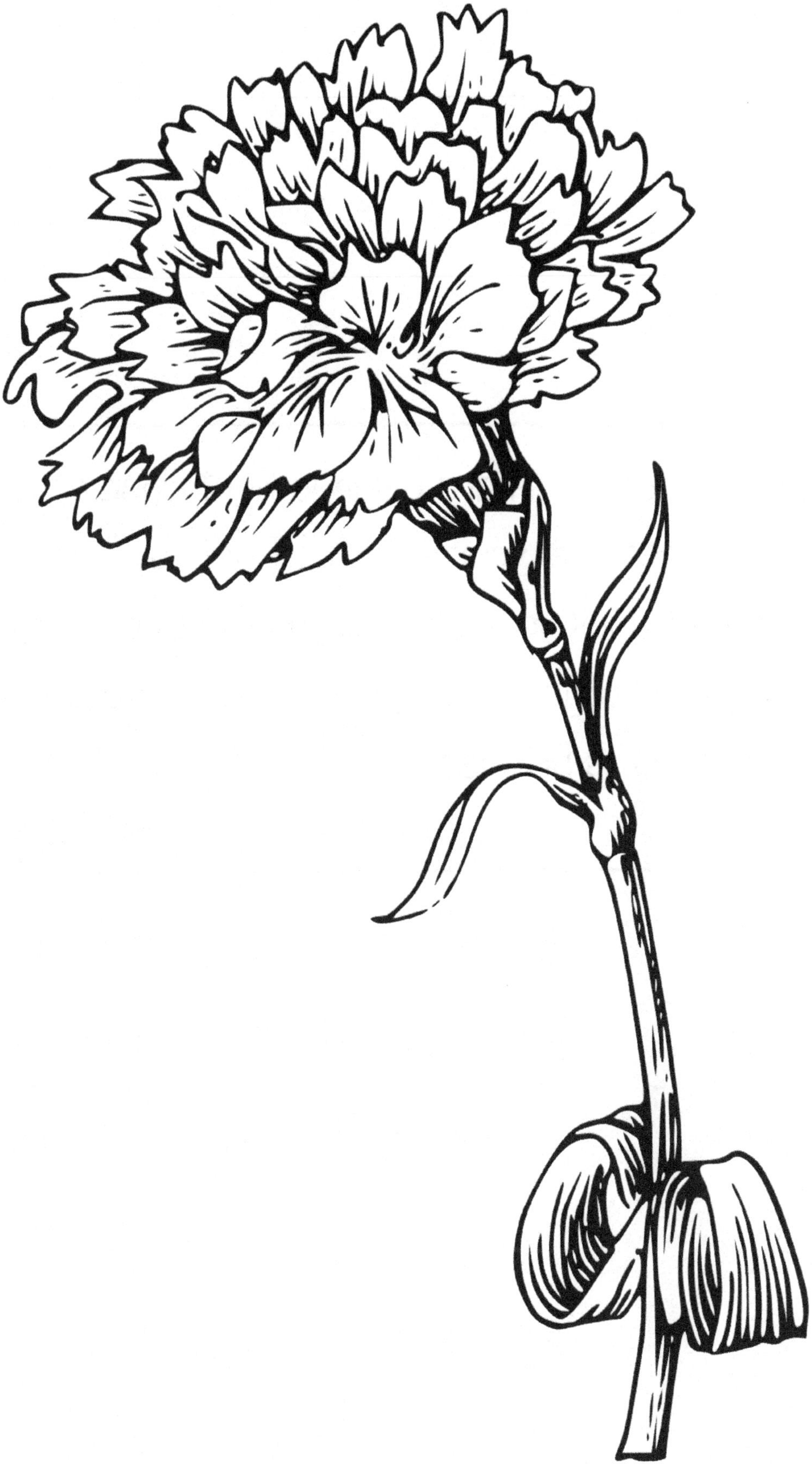

I think cancer is a hard battle to fight alone or with another person at your side, but I will say having someone to pick you up when you fall, stand by your side through every appointment and delivery of bad news, is priceless.

— Jenna Morasca

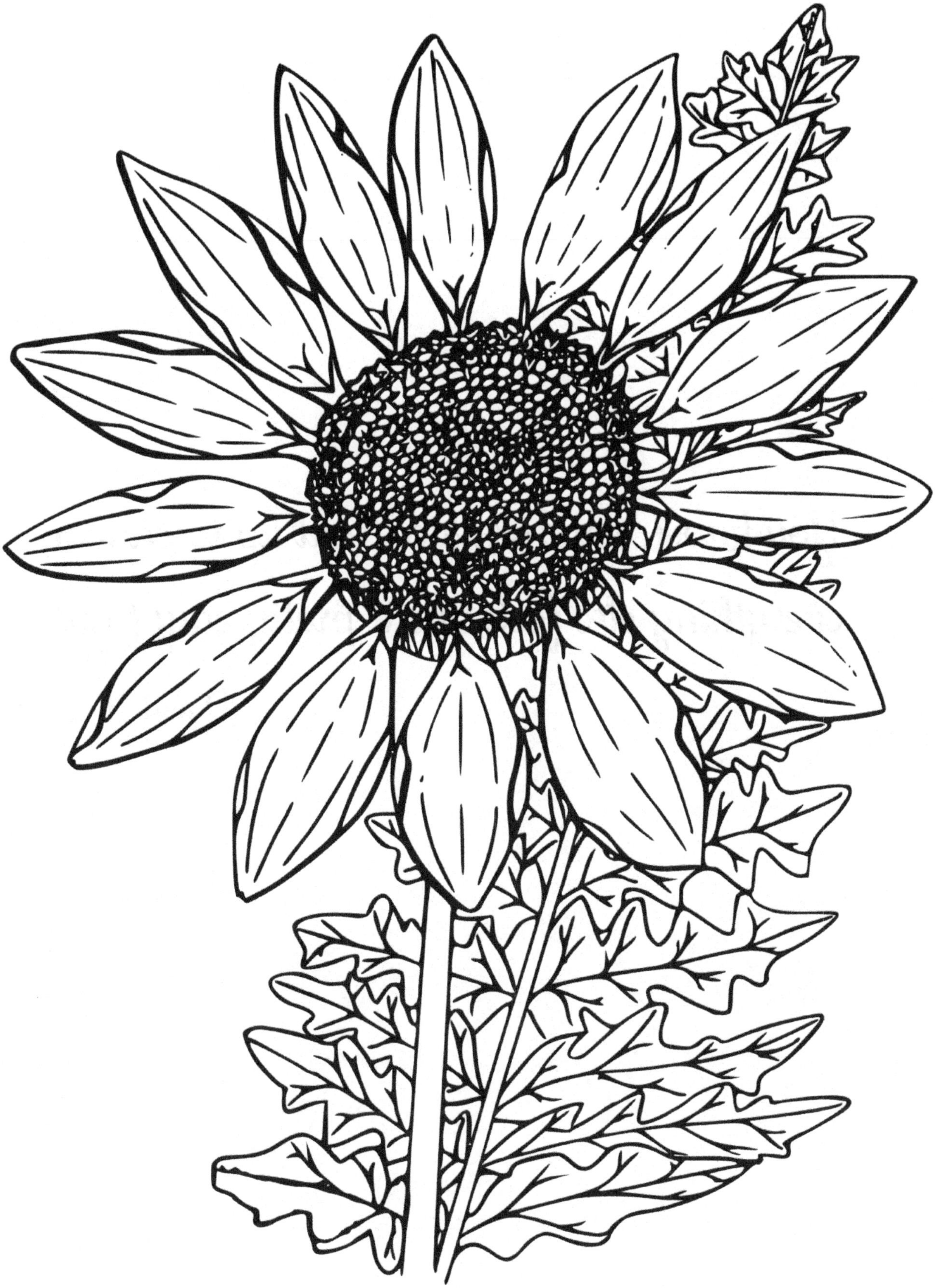

You know, once you've stood up to cancer,
everything else feels like a pretty easy fight.

– David H. Koch

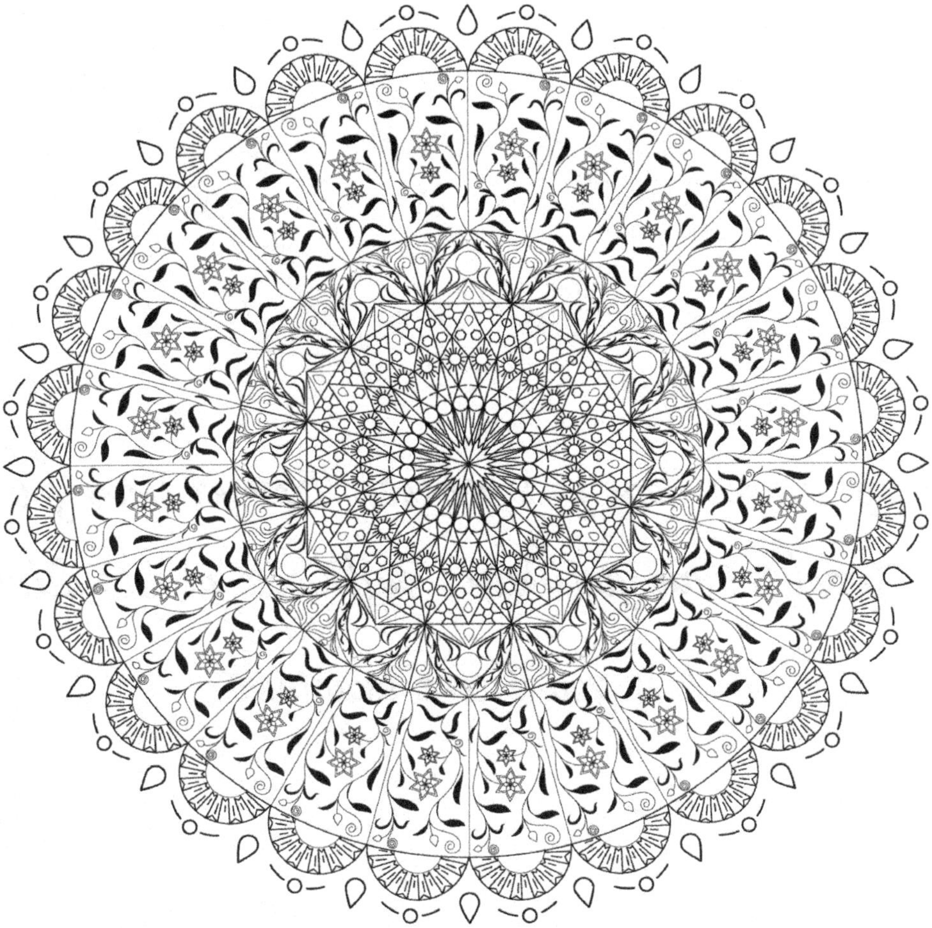

*You are braver than you believe, stronger than you seem,
smarter than you think, and twice as beautiful
as you'd ever imagined.*

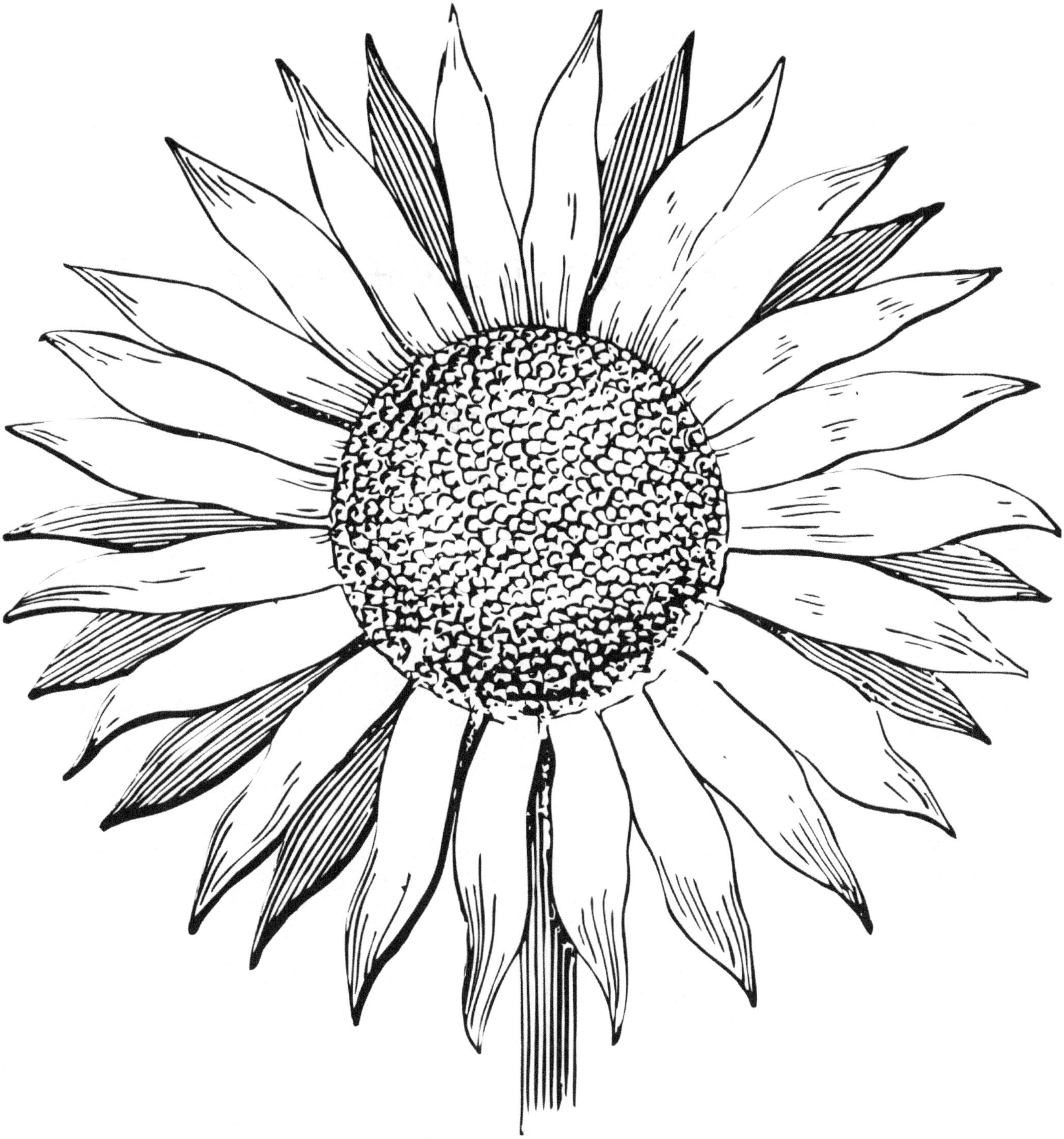

You can be a victim of cancer,
or a survivor of cancer.
It's a mindset.

– Dave Pelzer

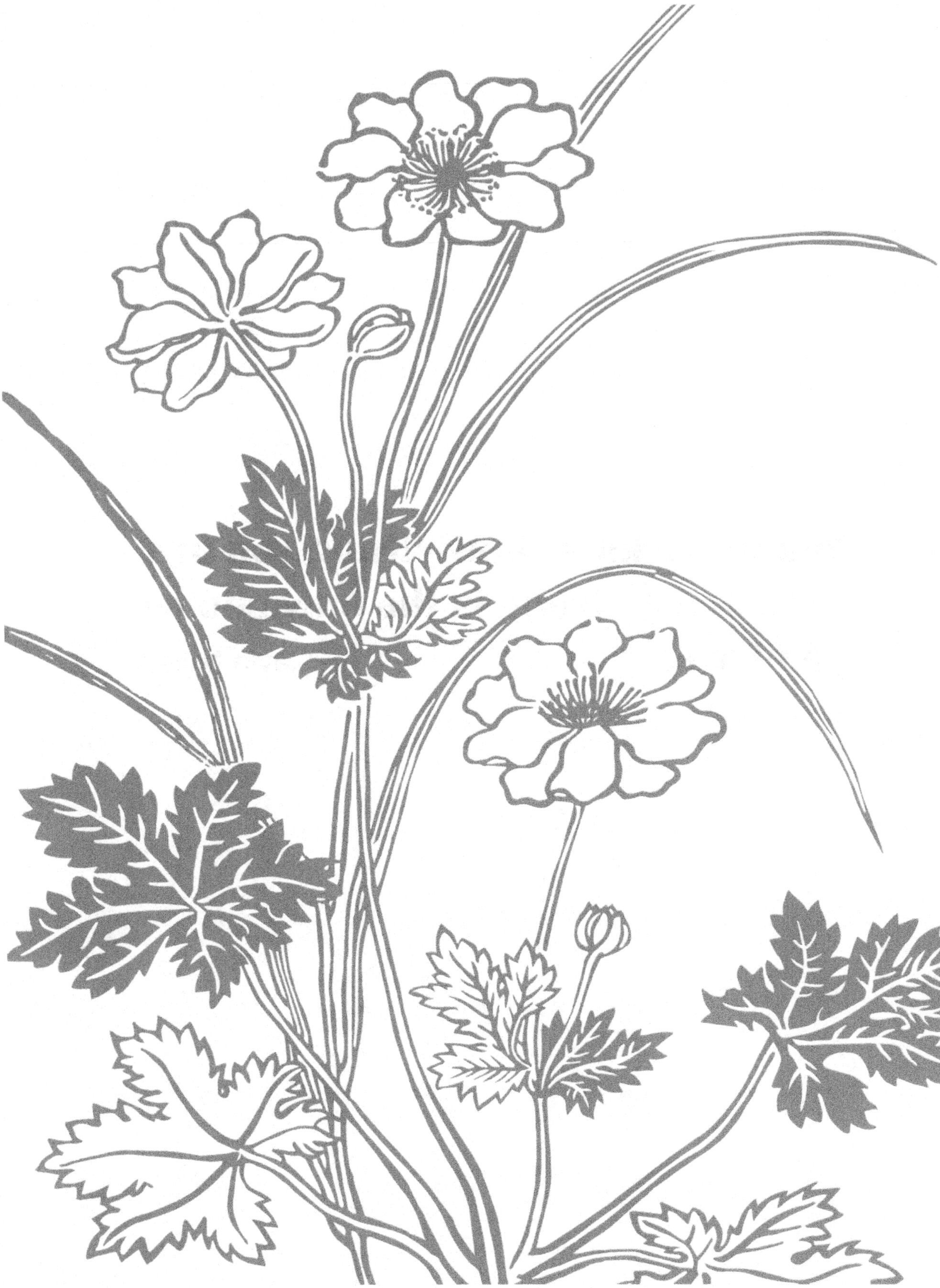

You never know how strong you are until being strong is the only choice you have. – Cayla Mills

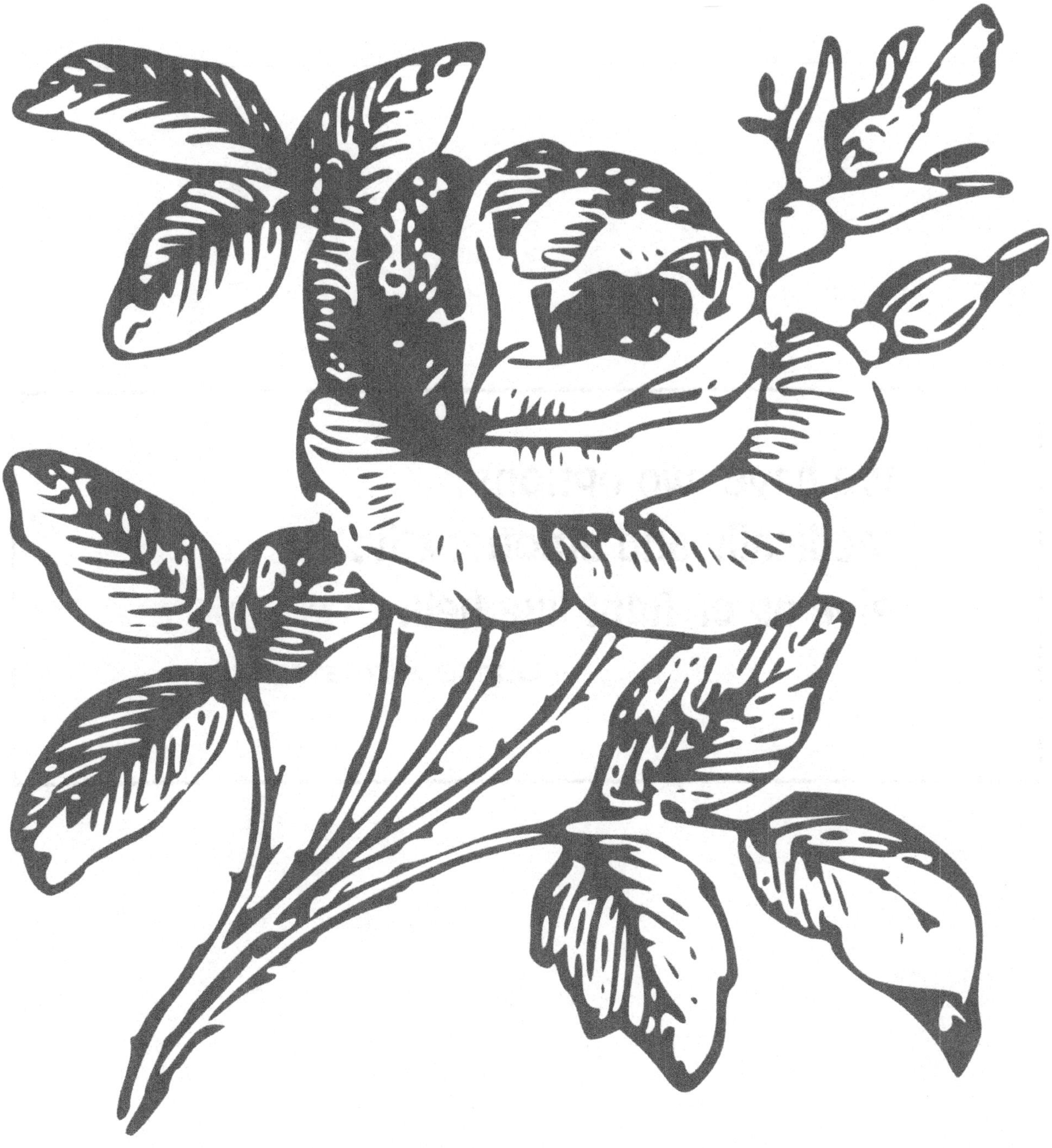

We have two options,
medically and emotionally:
give up or fight like hell.

- Lance Armstrong

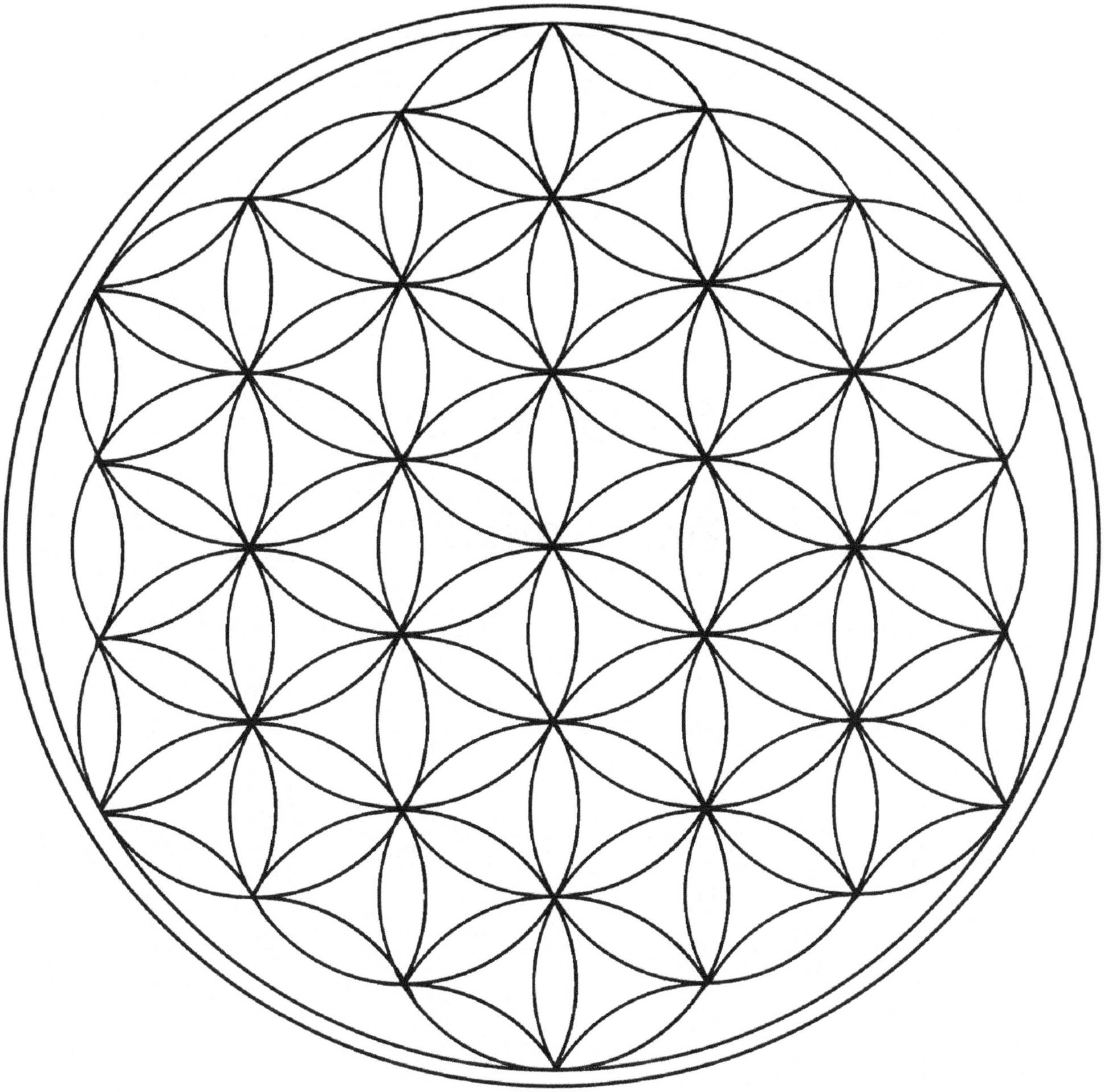

Small steps
every day.

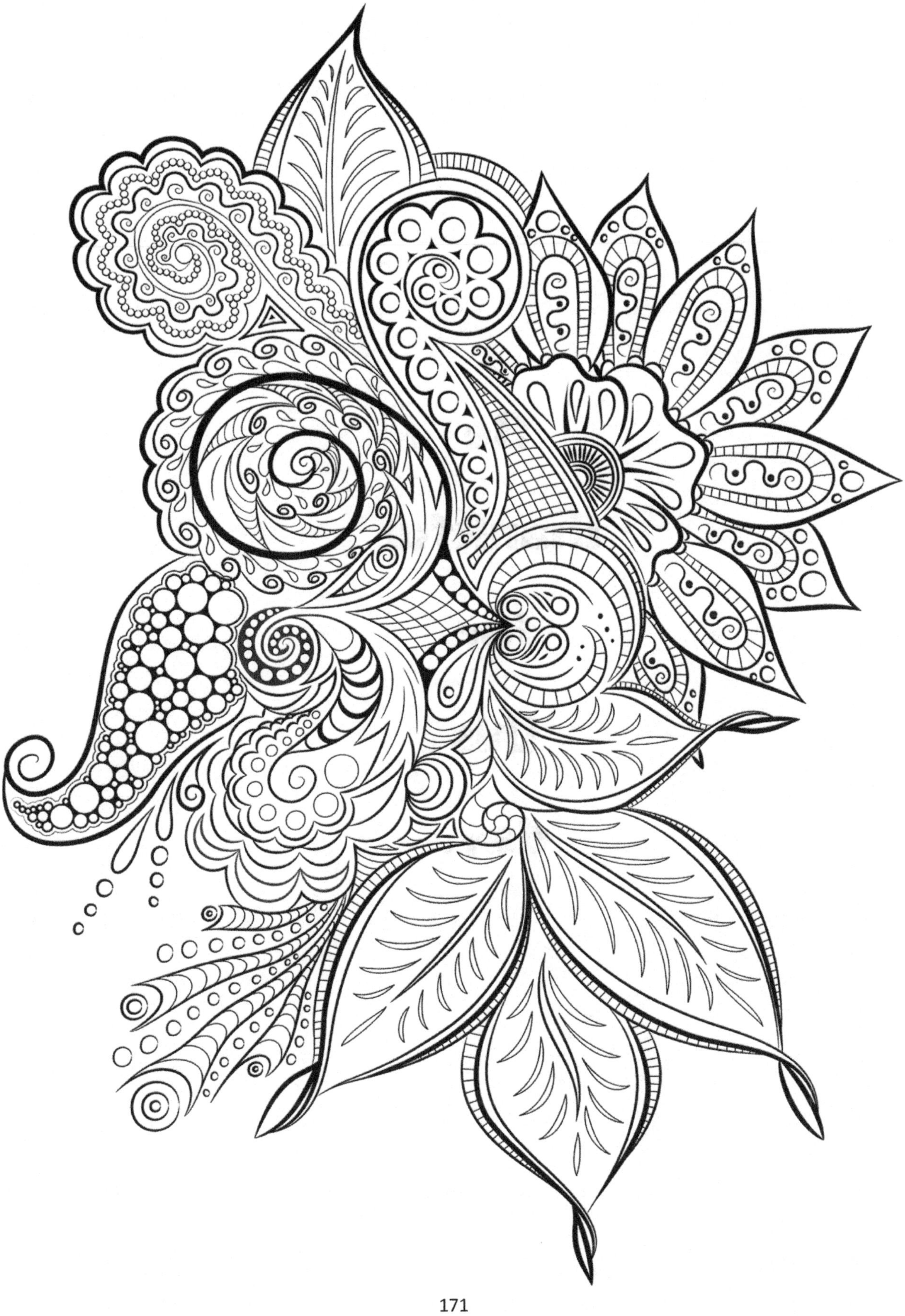

Be

thankful

for

this

day.

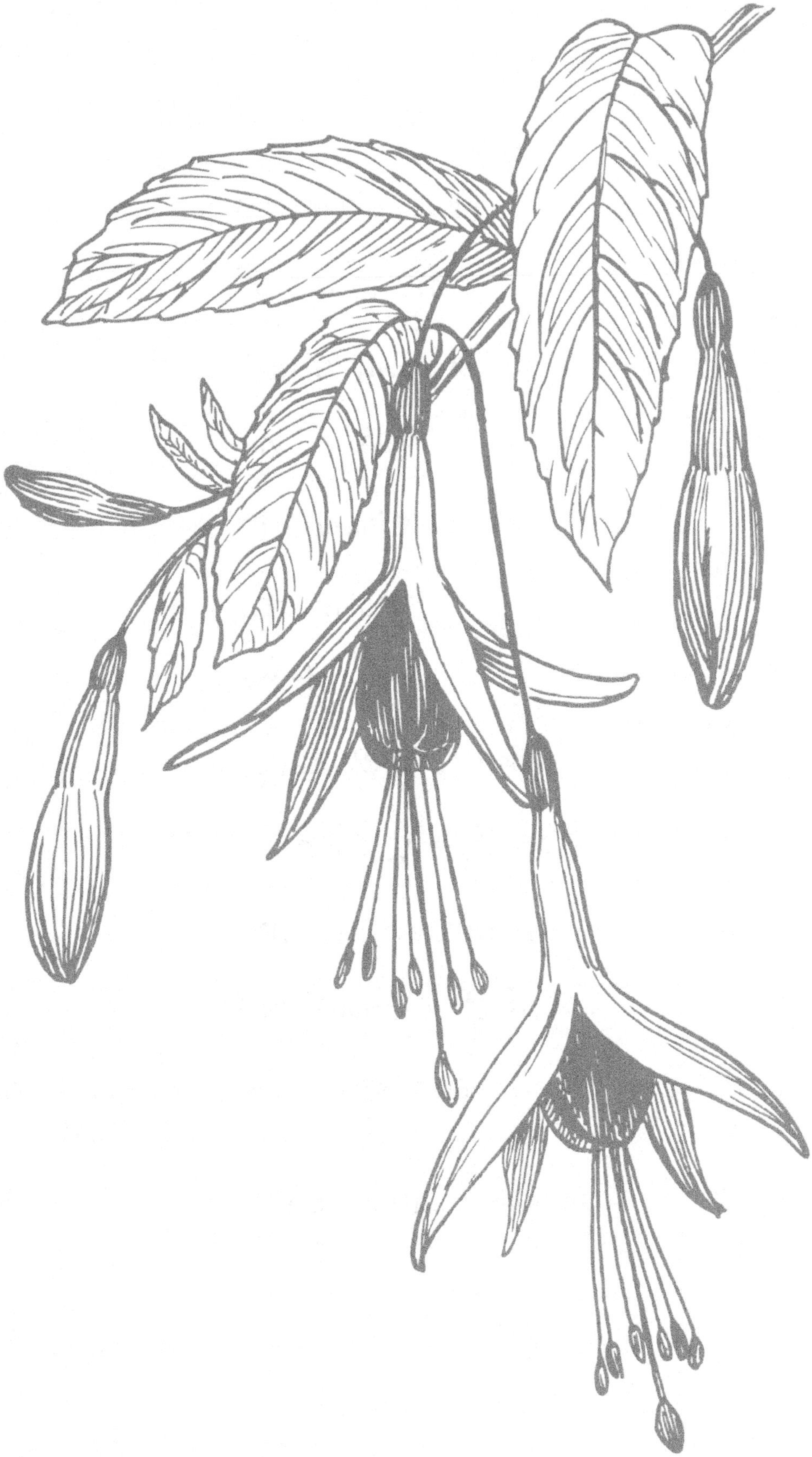

The ultimate
measure of
a man is not
where he
stands in
moments
of comfort
and convenience,
but where he
stands at a time
of challenge and
controversy.

– Dr. Martin Luther King Jr.

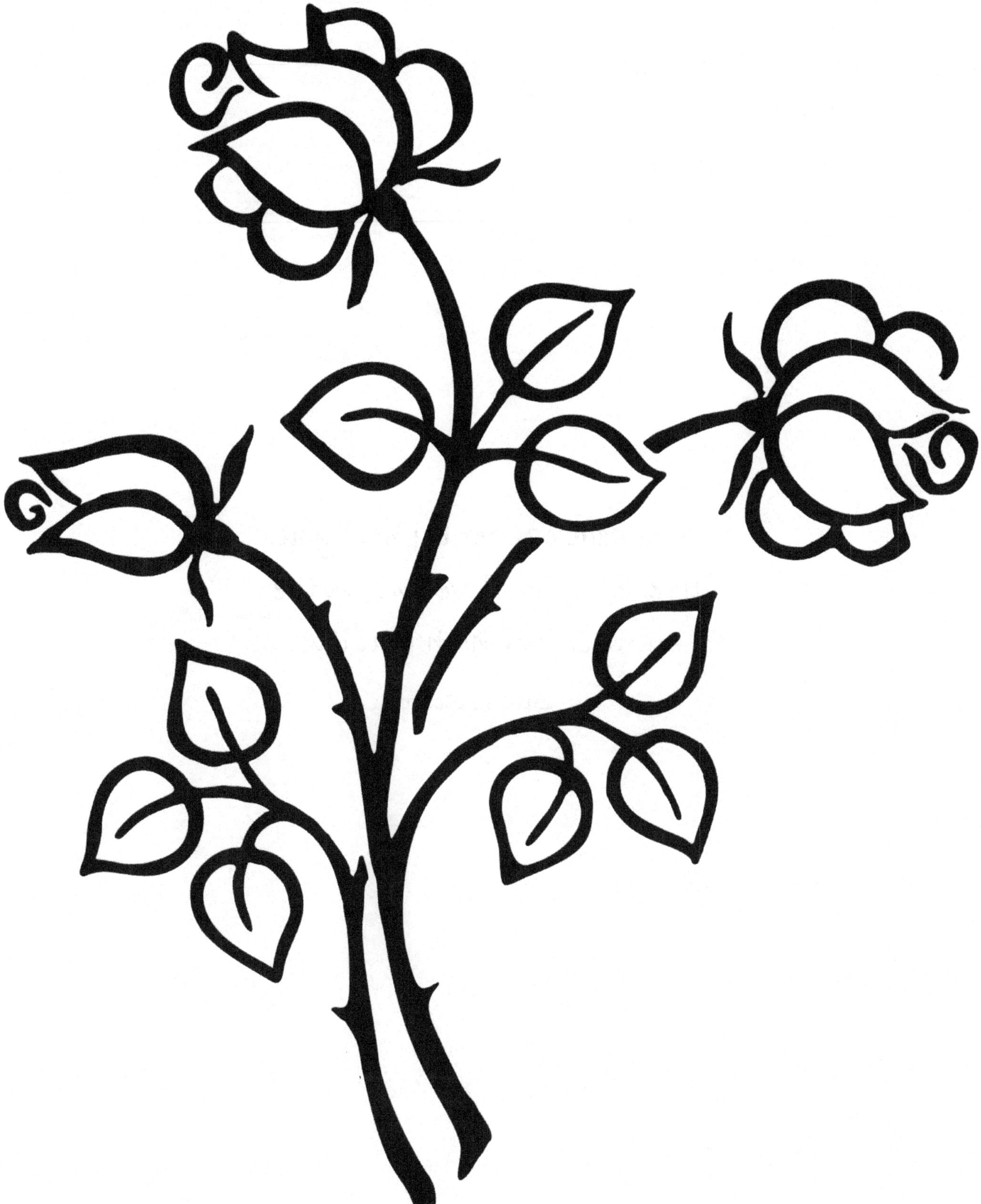

You beat cancer by how you live, why you live and in the manner in which you live.

– Stuart Scott

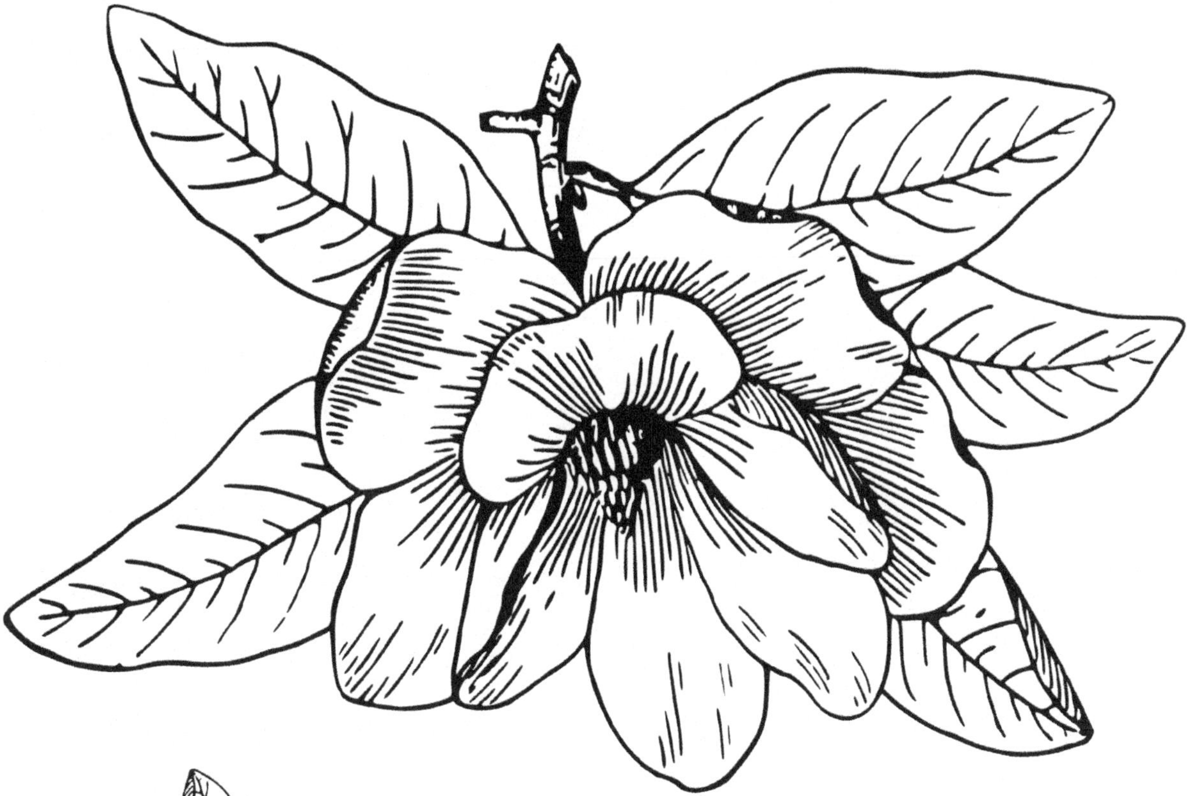

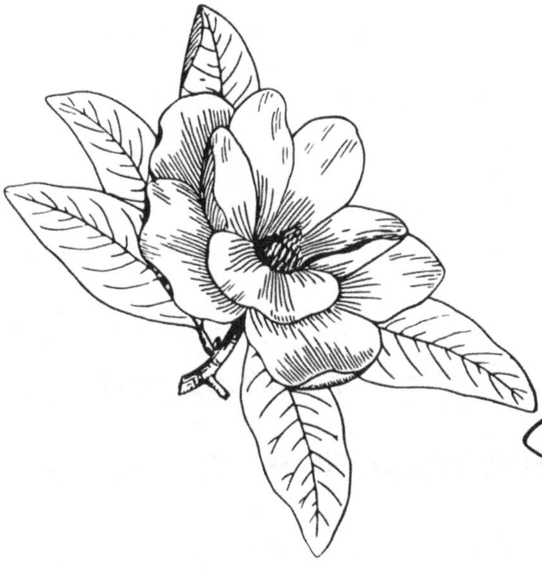

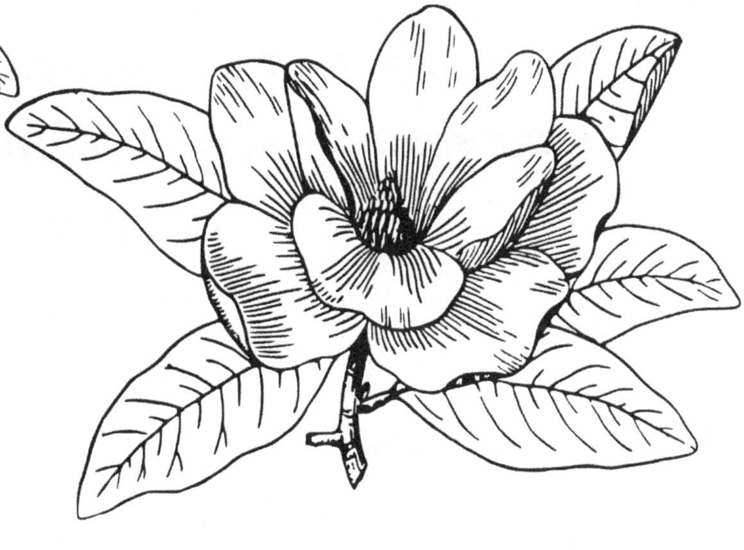

NEVER BE ASHAMED OF A SCAR. IT SIMPLY MEANS YOU WERE STRONGER THAN WHATEVER TRIED TO HURT YOU.

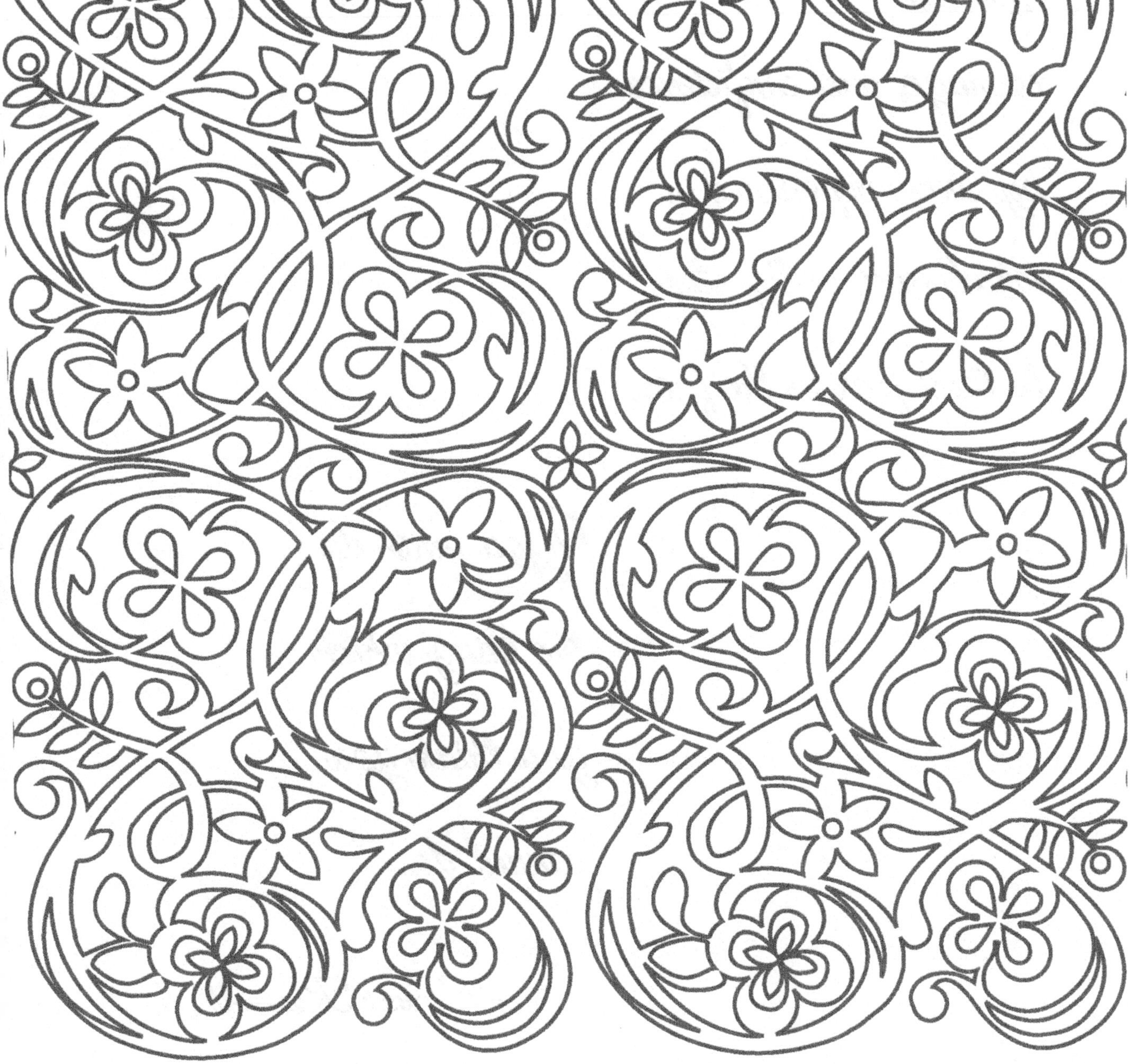

You gain strength,
courage, and confidence
by every experience in
which you really stop
to look fear in the face.

You must do
the thing which
you think you
cannot do.

– Eleanor Roosevelt

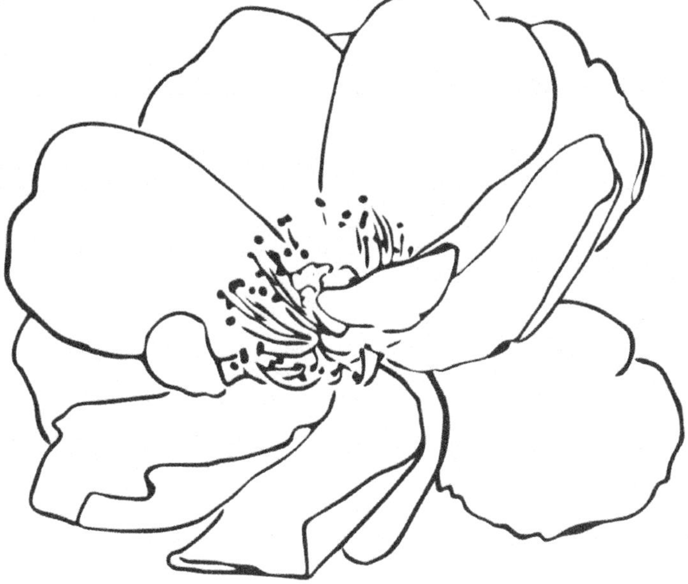

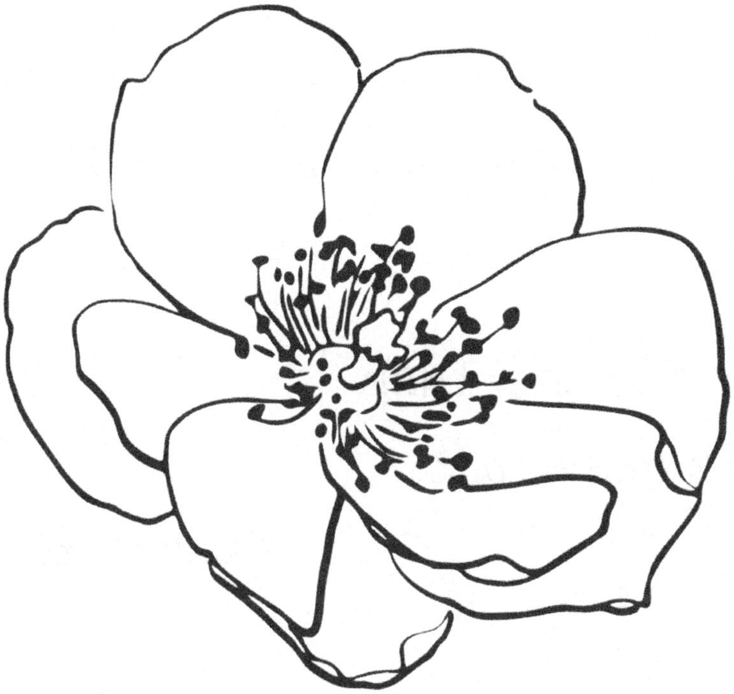

The human spirit is stronger than anything that can happen to it.

– C.C. Scott

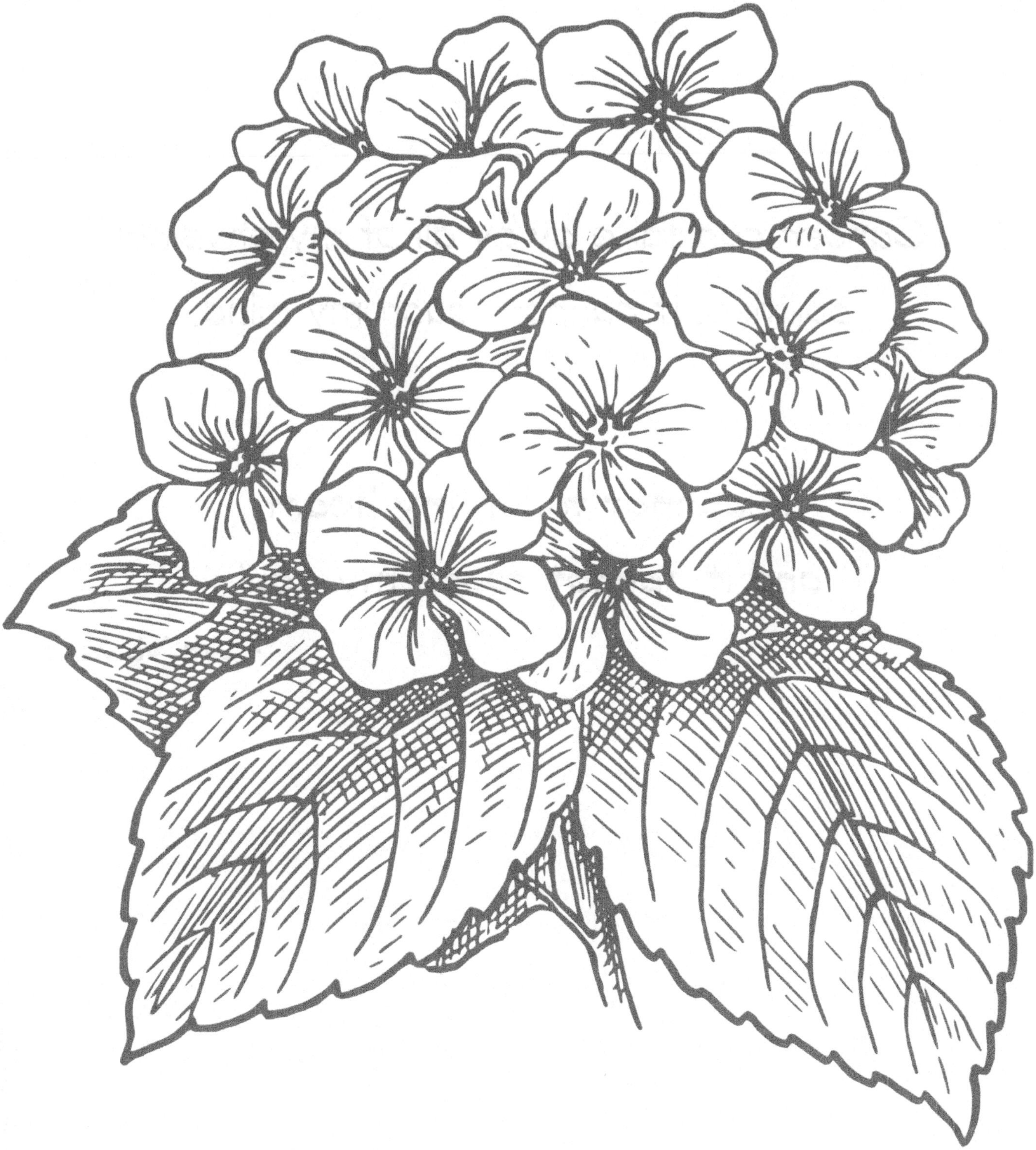

Cancer can take away all of my physical abilities. It cannot touch my mind,

it cannot touch my heart,
and it cannot touch my soul.

- Jim Valvano

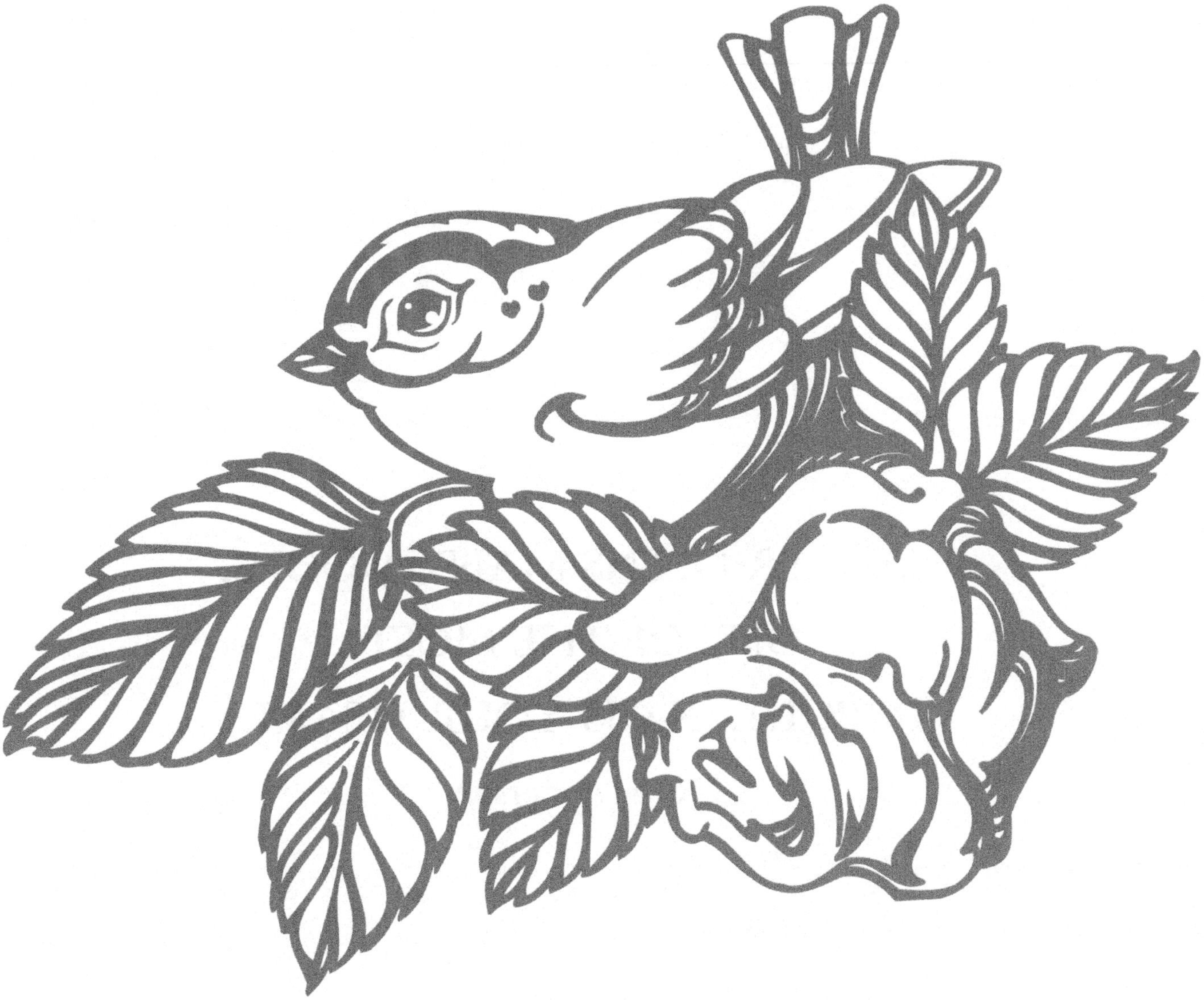

CANCER OPENS MANY DOORS.
ONE OF THE MOST
IMPORTANT IS YOUR HEART.

– Greg Anderson

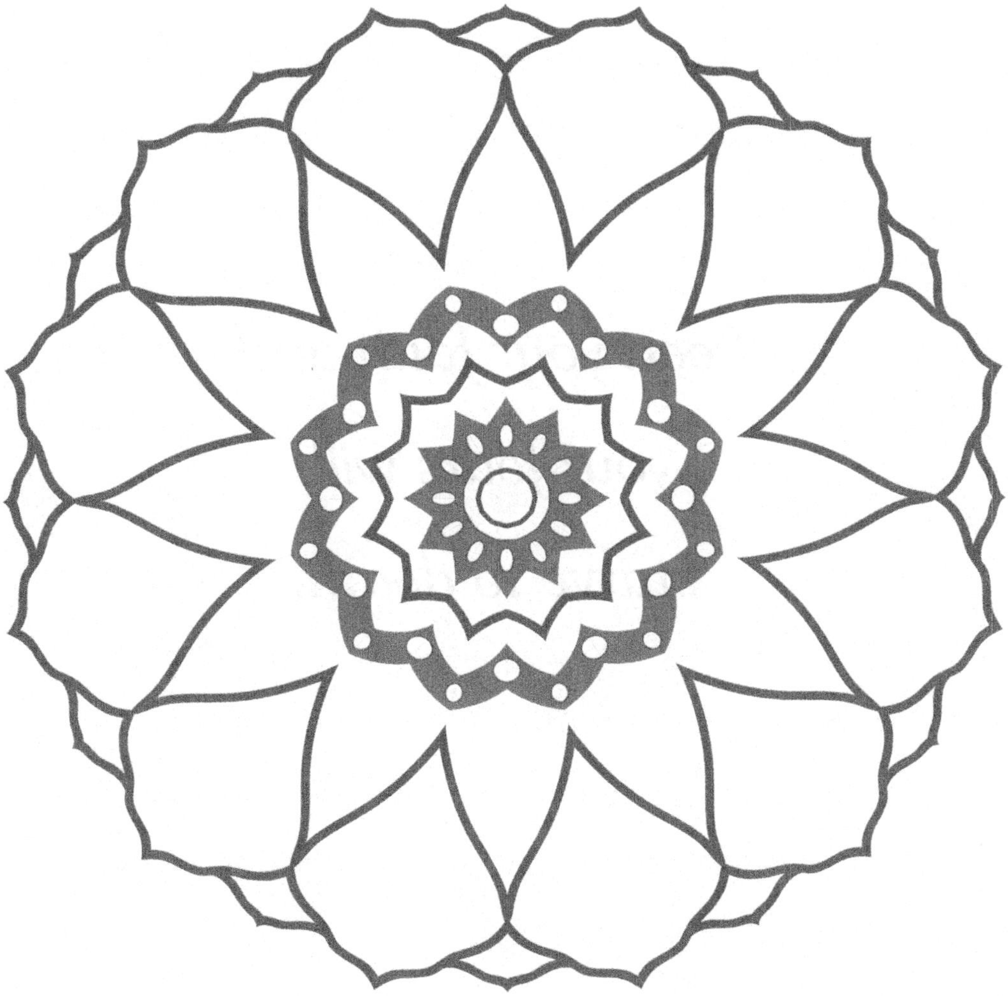

Feed your faith and

your fears will

starve to death.

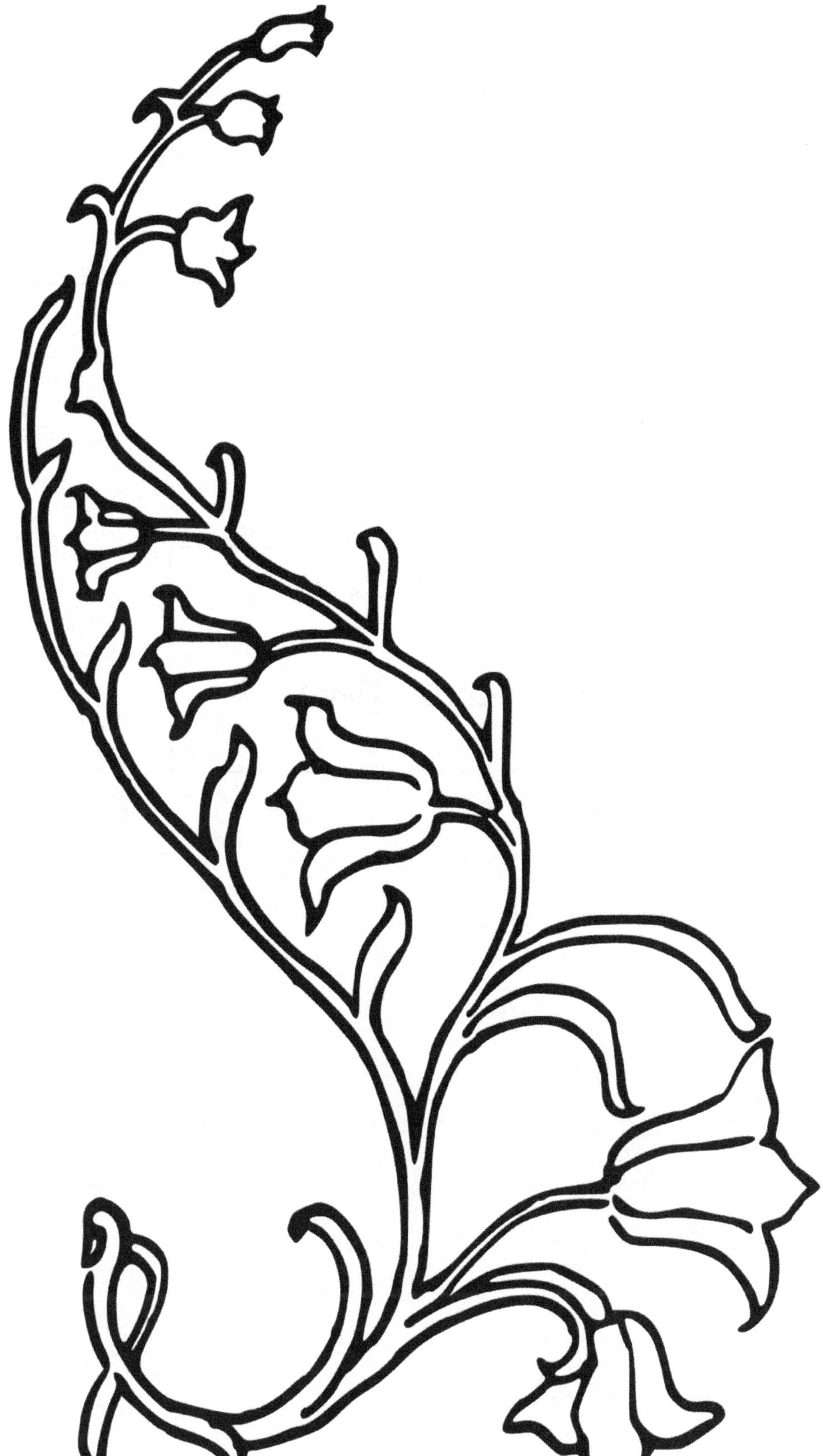

I had cancer.

Cancer <u>never</u> had me.

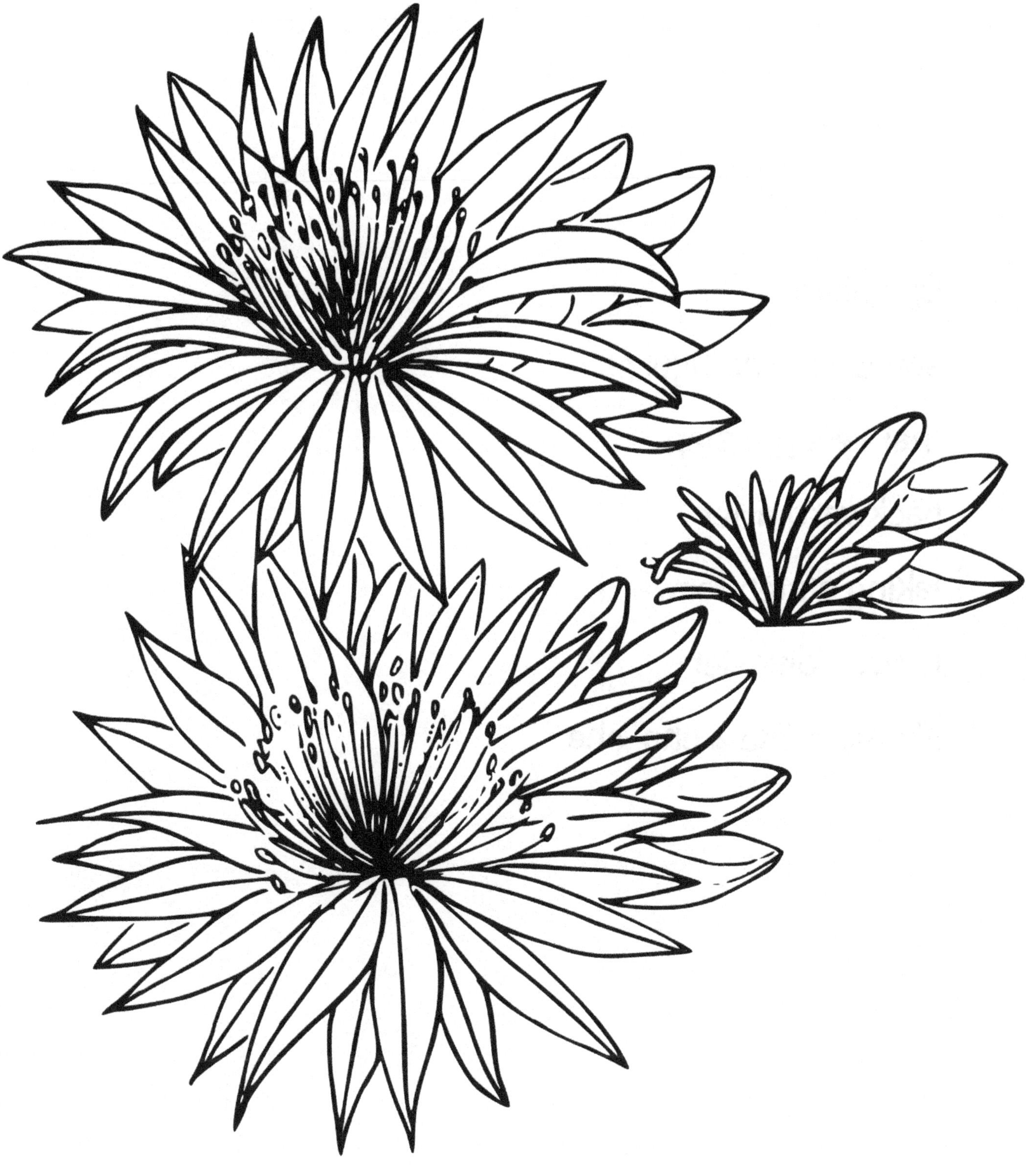

Optimism:

someone who figures
that taking a step
backward after
taking a step forward
is not a disaster;
it's more like a cha-cha.

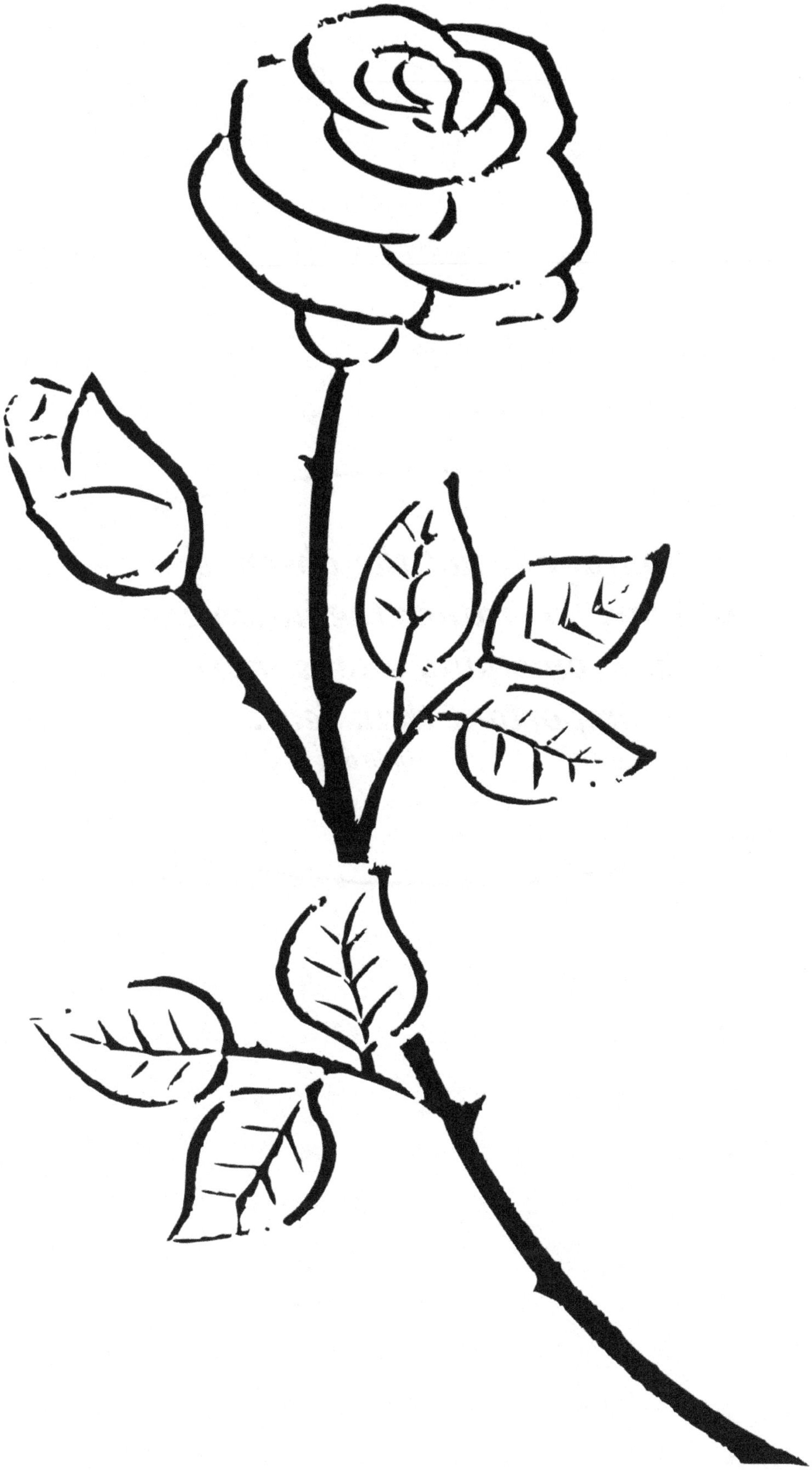

Courage is not the absence of fear, but rather the judgment that something else is more important than fear.

- Ambrose Redmoon

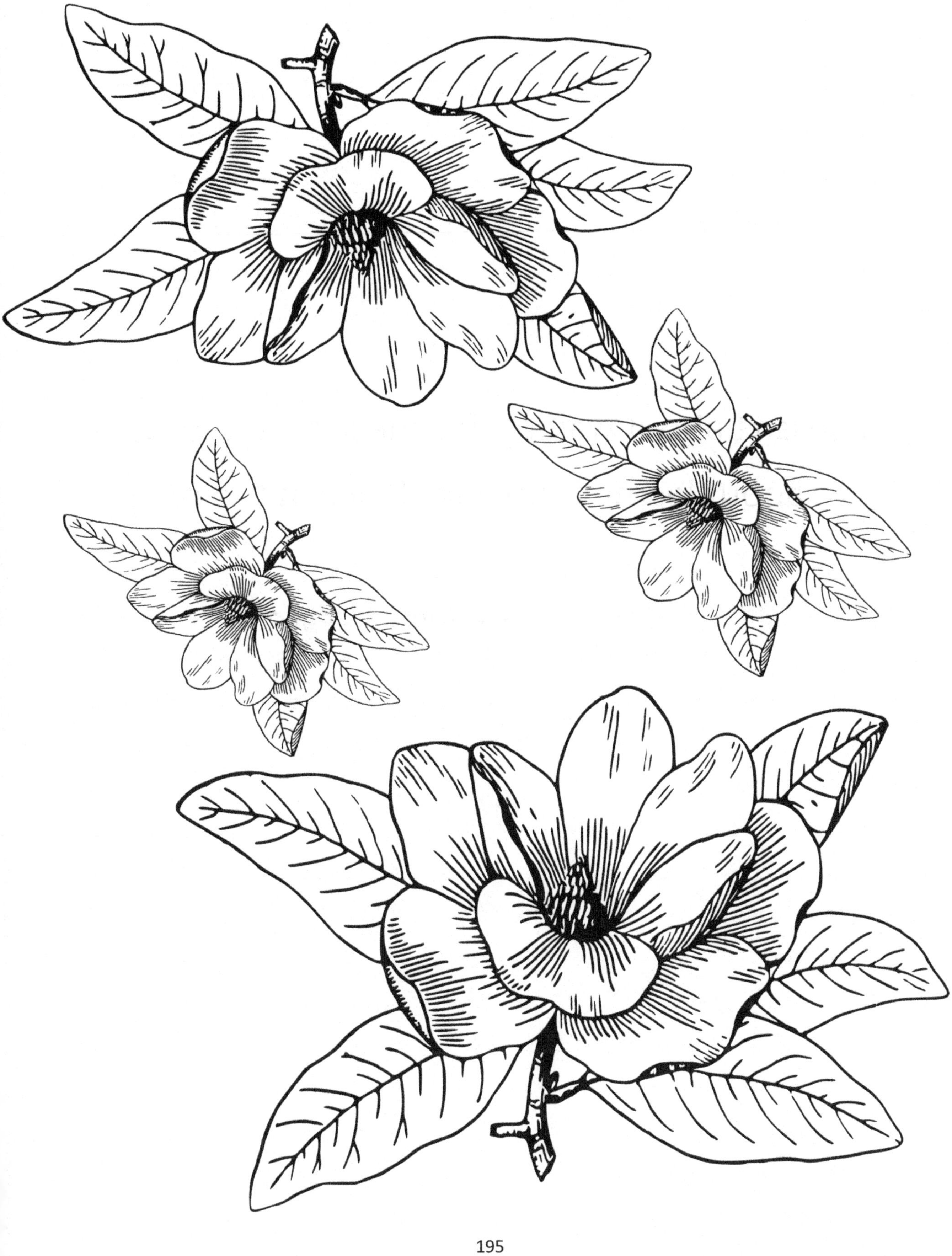

Life isn't about waiting for the storm to pass,

it's about learning how to dance in the rain.

- Lindsay Hodgson

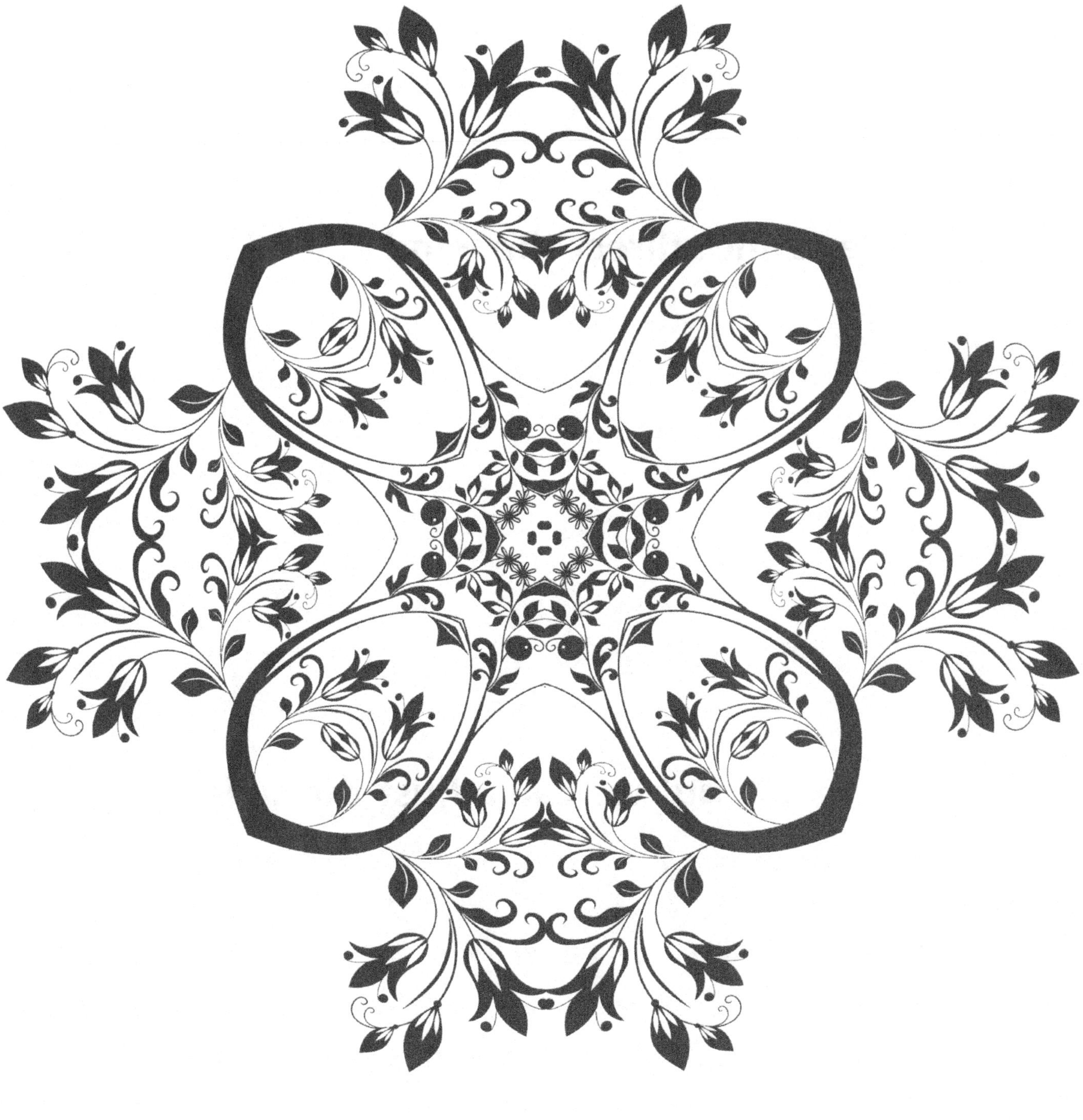

We cannot direct the wind . . .

. . . but we can adjust the sails.

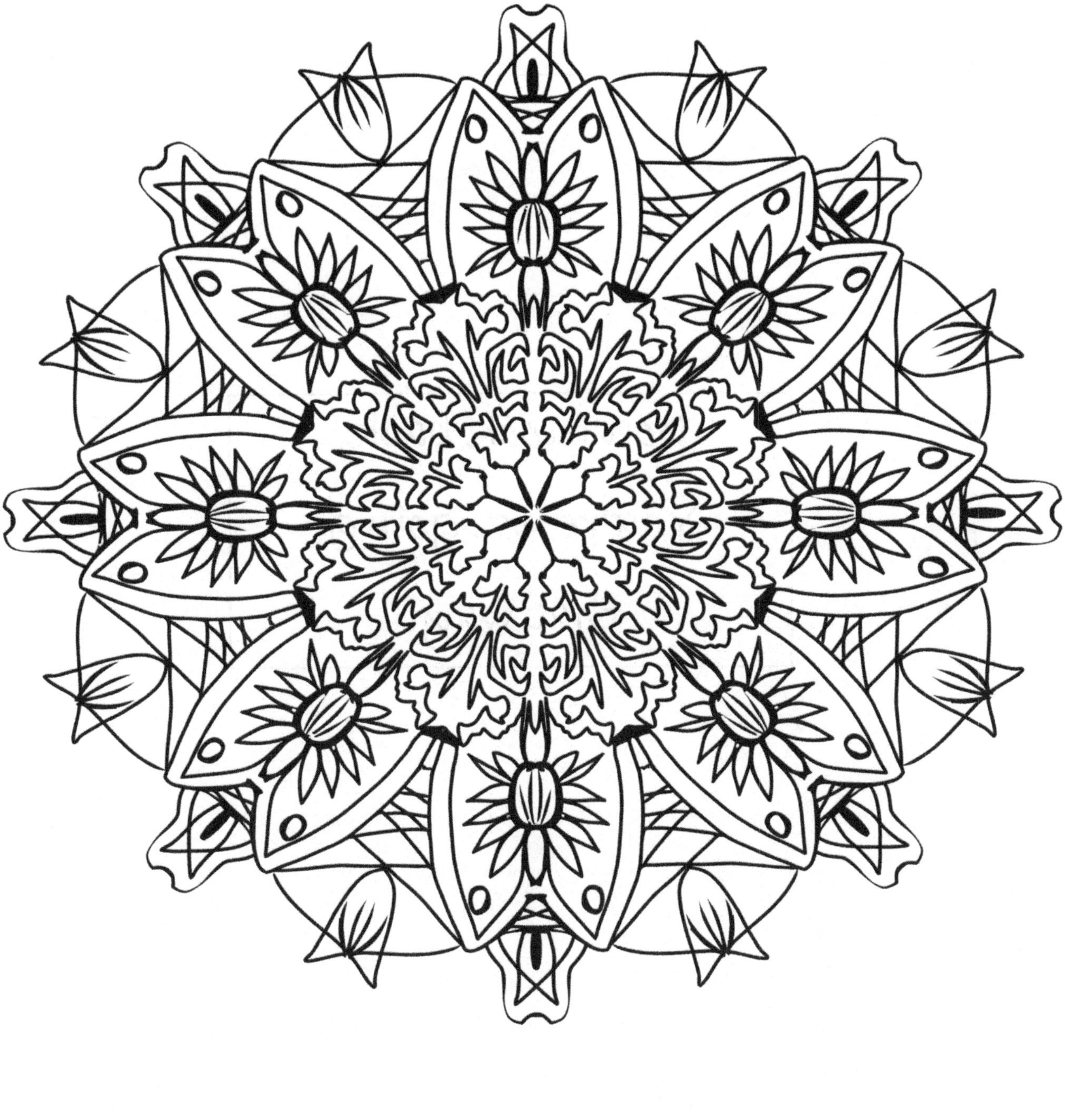

Don't look back.

You're not going

that way.

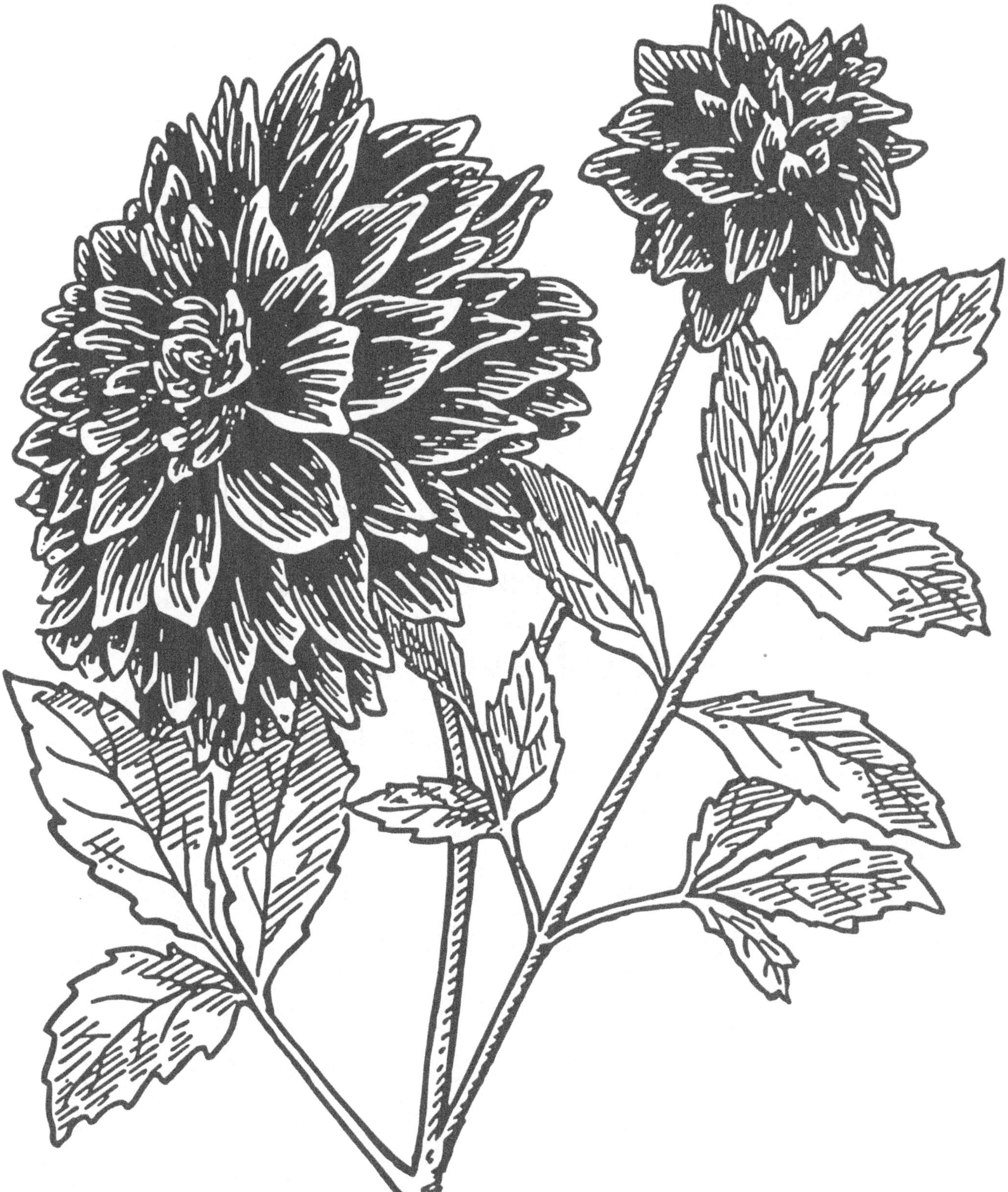

When you have exhausted all possibilities, remember this:

You haven't.

– Thomas Edison

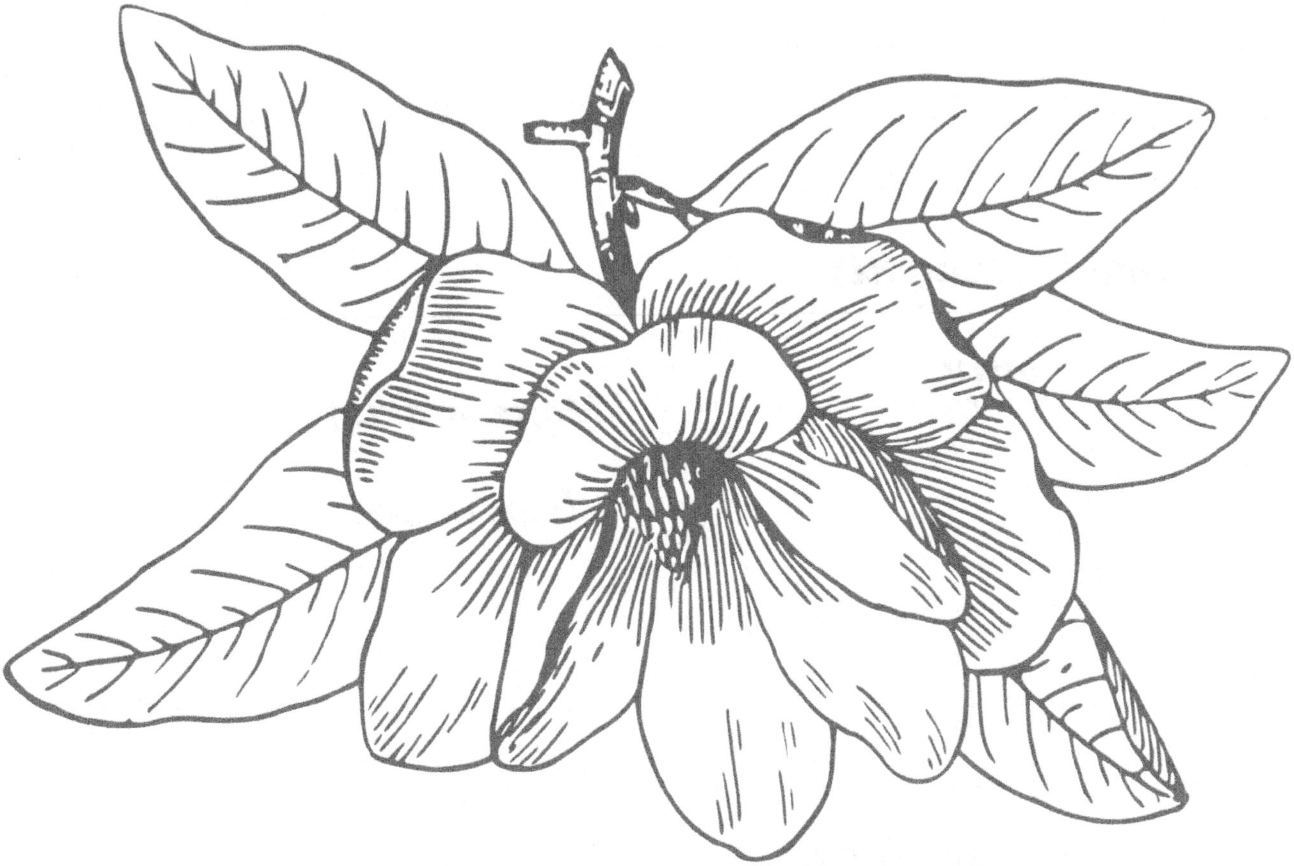

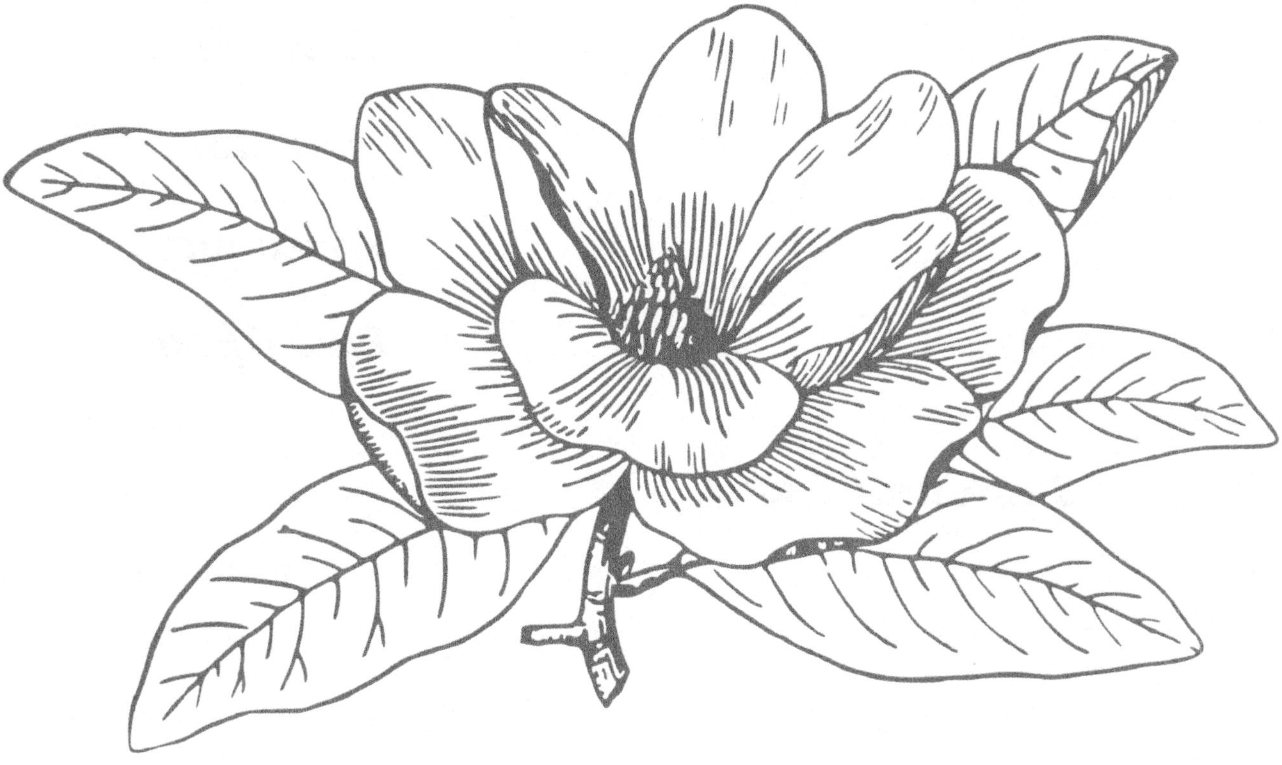

Good . thoughts .
only.

Hope is grief's
best music.

Never give up.
Never give in.

Your life is
your story.
Write well.
Edit Often.

I can and I will.

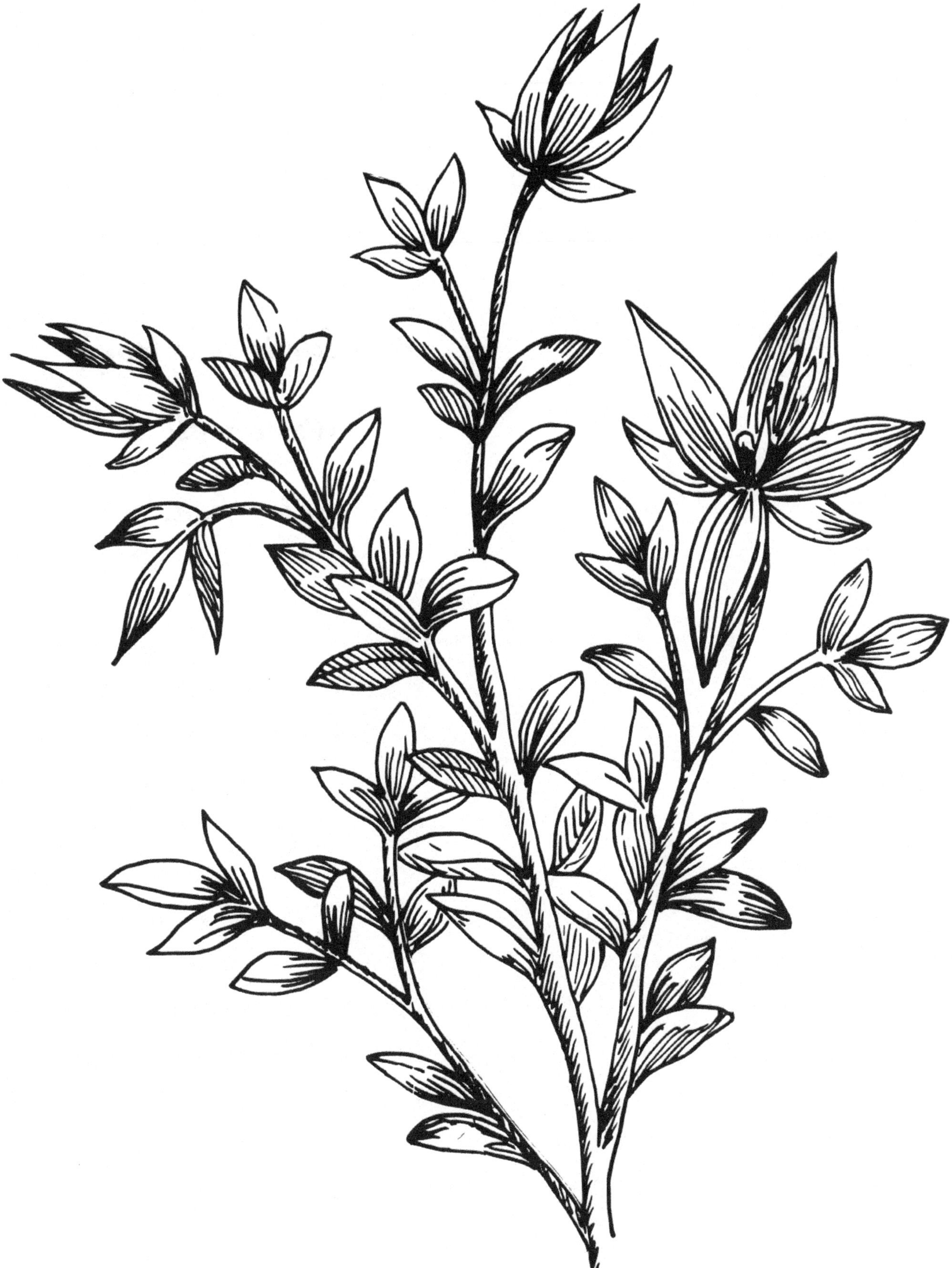

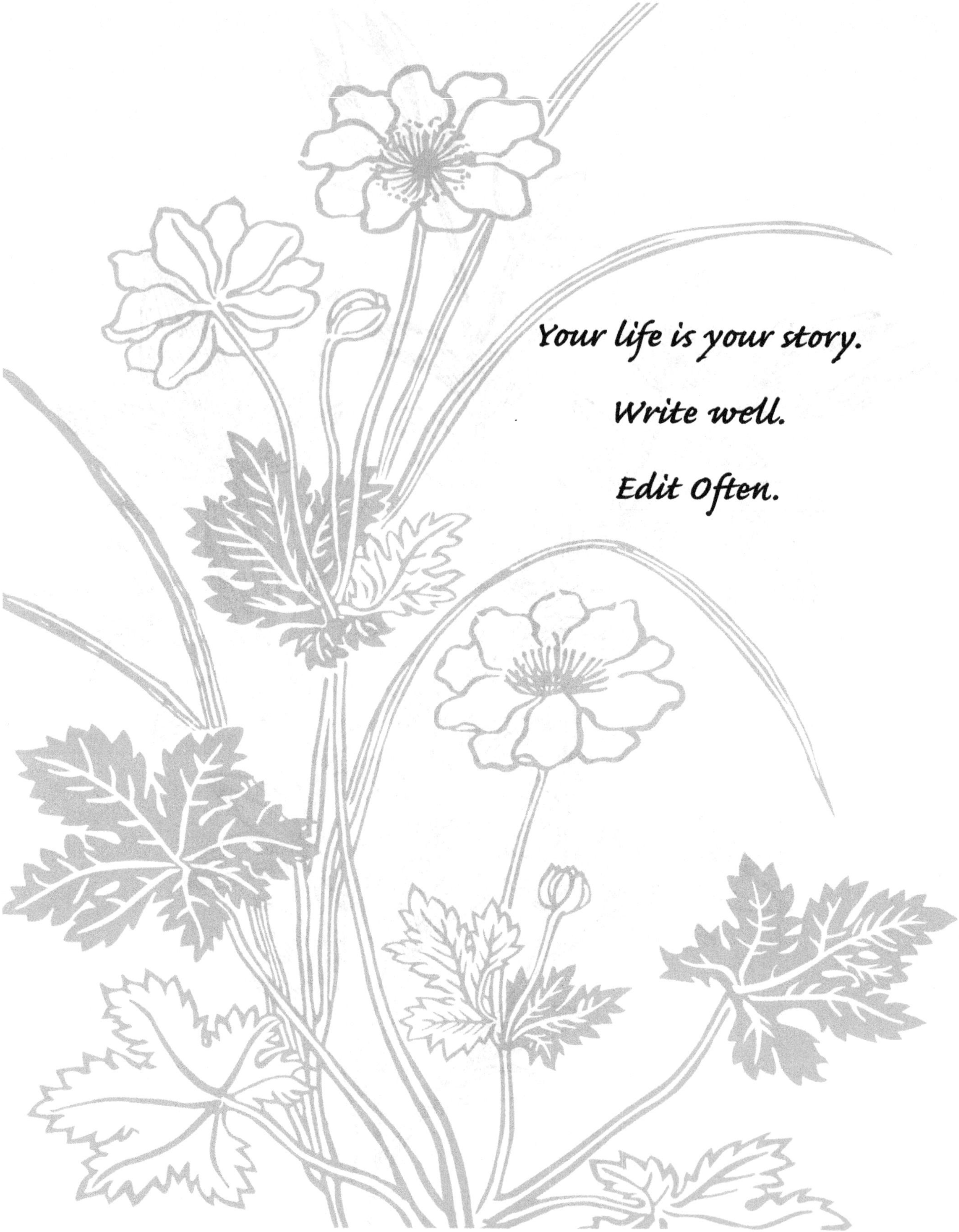

Your life is your story.

Write well.

Edit Often.

Other books available by the author on Amazon

Journals

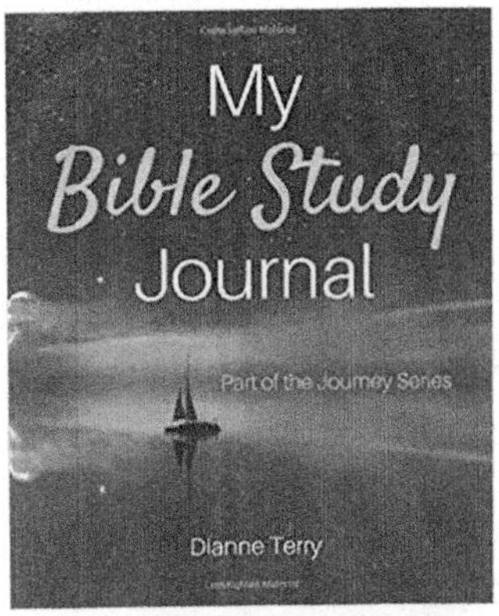

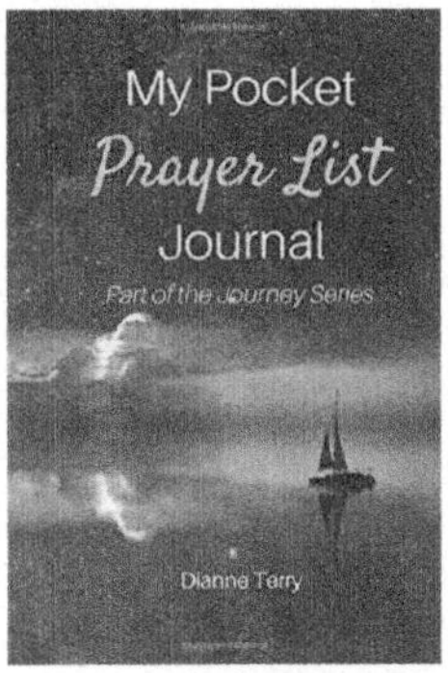

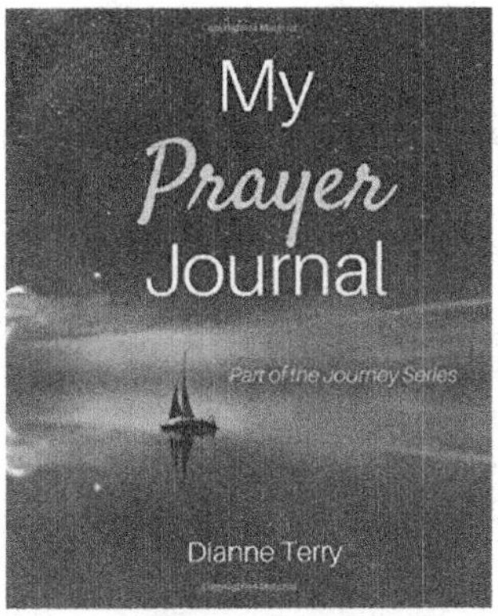

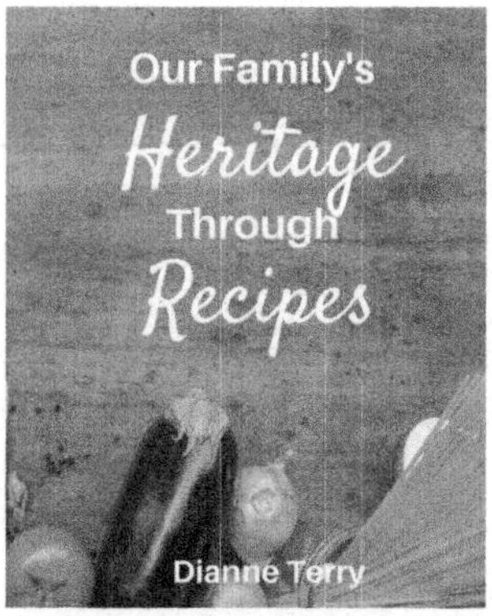

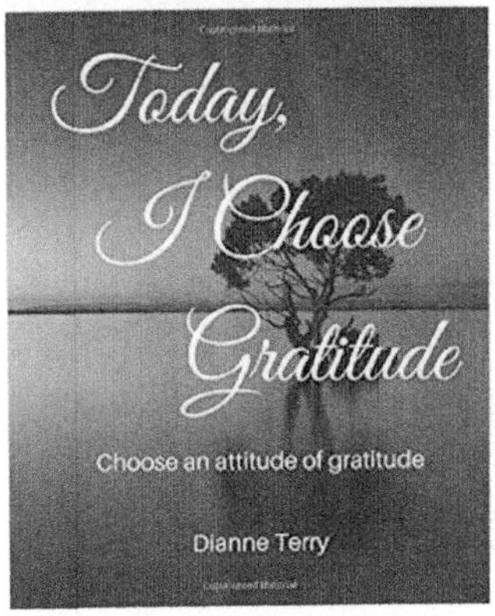

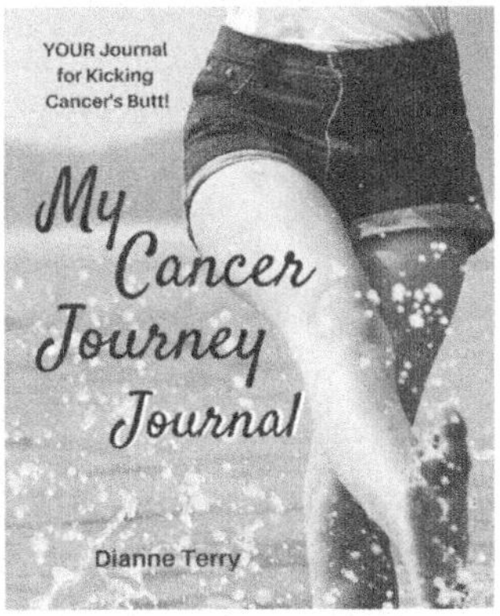

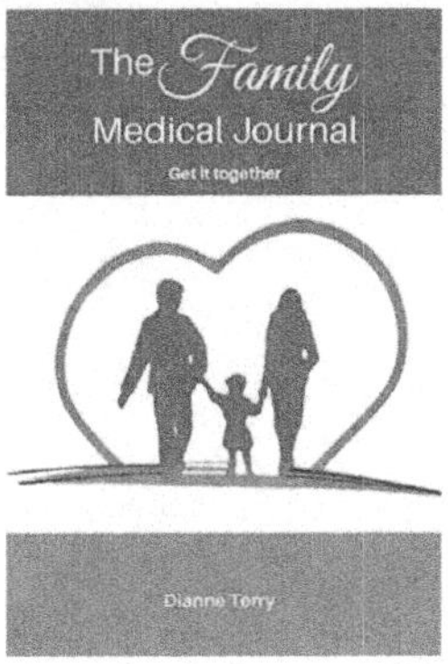

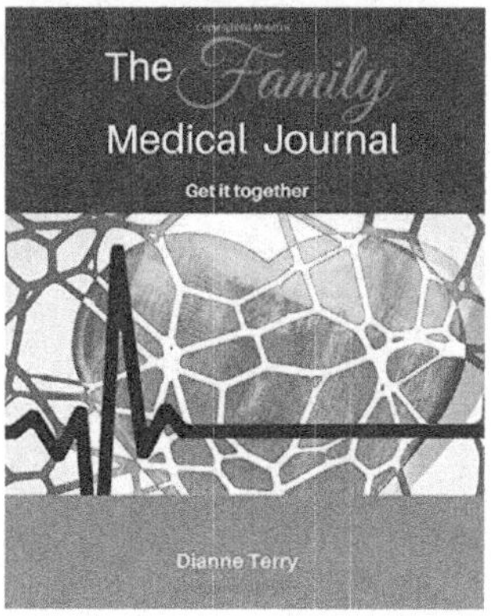

Gift Books

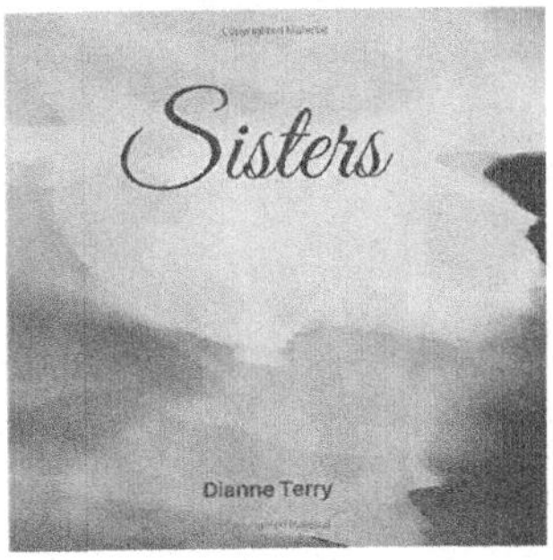

eBook and Paperback

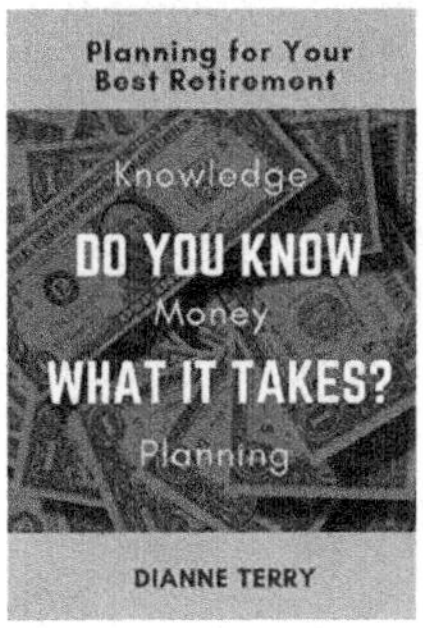

Made in the USA
Monee, IL
05 November 2026

67380094R00116